RECLAIM YOUR HEALTH

A GUIDE TO

REDISCOVERING

YOUR INNER HEALER

Dr. James W Zielinski DC

Important Information For the Reader

This information presented in this book has been compiled from my clinical experience and research. It is offered as a view of the relationship between diet, exercise, emotions, and health. This book is not intended for, self diagnosis or treatment of disease, nor is it a substitute for the advice and care of a licensed health care provider. Sharing of the information in this book with the attending physician is highly desirable.

This book is intended solely to help you make better judgements concerning your long-term health goals. If you are experiencing health problems, you should consult a qualified physician immediately. Remember early examination and detection are important to successful treatment of all diseases.

Table Of Contents

CHAPTER 1

The Opioid Epidemic Of The United States

As per the data provided by the CDC, mortality related to the abuse of opioids remains the major health issue in the united states. The opioid nightmare is the primary reason for drug-related deaths, accounting for almost 60% of deaths due to a drug overdose. Since 1999 the number of deaths related to drug overdoses have risen by four, these numbers include overdoses both due to prescription medications and heroin. If we look at the figures of the total number of deaths happening, it is truly alarming. Every day almost 91 Americans are dying due to opioid overdose, thus between 2000-2015 more than half a million US residents have been killed because of it[1].

Thus the question arises, what is behind this rising problem? The answer to this question is even more worrisome. It is the prescription opioid and not the street drugs that are behind this whole issue, something pretty obvious from the statistics. Prescription of opioids has risen by four times between the period of 1999-2010. It is troublesome, considering the fact that painful conditions among the US population have not increased at that pace, in fact, they have not risen much over the decade.

However, use of prescription painkillers is reaching staggering numbers. It is no more a controversy that their usage has taken the form of an epidemic in the US. This epidemic has been fueled by the vast number of factors in the prescription drug system.

"Calm mind brings inner strength and self-confidence, so that's very important for good health."

Dalai Lama

So what is the abuse of a prescription drug? Well, it is the use of prescription drugs for unapproved reasons, not just for pain relief, but for their psychoactive properties or use of prescription drugs for recreation. Although this is in no way a new problem, what is genuinely new is the alarming upsurge in the abuse.

The medical community and its stakeholders are already accepting the fact that the problem exists, and that patients are virtually "doctor shopping," trying to find the doctors that will prescribe the opioids. Further, the scientific community, healthcare system, the pharmaceutical industry, and regulatory bodies have manipulated data. These factors have led to the problem that we are witnessing today.

To further understand the gravity of the problem, consider the fact that 16 million US residents reported using at least one prescription drug during the last year. An overwhelming number of them stated that they had taken prescription drugs during the previous one month[2].

Not to say that all of the use of prescription medications is harmful, but this does highlight the over-prescription of such drugs. When used for the intended purpose, prescription drugs can bring a level of relief and quality of life when the pain is otherwise unresponsive to treatment, however, many of the medications prescribed are addictive in nature, and their abuse, can lead to serious health issues, and in some cases may be fatal.

"To enjoy good health, to bring true happiness to one's family, to bring peace to all, one must first discipline and control one's own mind. If a man can control his mind he can find the way to Enlightenment, and all wisdom and virtue will naturally come to him".

Buddha

In 2010, a national survey brought to the forefront the dangerous trend of abuse of prescription drugs. As per the report, around seven million Americans were using psychoactive prescription medications for the purpose other than intended. That means that at any given time at least 3% of Americans are abusing prescription drugs. The most commonly used drugs were painkillers, as pain is subjective and cannot be substatianted or unsubstantiated with objective testing. Figures indicate 5.1 million users, followed by 1.1 million users of psychostimulants, and another 0.4 Americans for sedatives[2].

Equally worrying are the figures regarding the use of prescription medications among adolescents, considering that their nervous system is still developing and making them more prone to addiction. Between 2010 to 2011 almost one in twelve high school aged adolescents were reported to be taking Vicodin, for non-medical reasons and one in 20 high school seniors were regularly abusing the highly addictive painkiller OxyContin.

Research also demonstrated a loophole in the system, considering the ease with which high school seniors were able to obtain these highly regulated medications. In the survey, most of them reported that they received those drugs from either relatives or friends.

Therefore it should be no surprise when data from CDC show that almost more than 90 Americans are dying each day due to opioid overuse, and the majority of these deaths are a result of prescription opiods. Data from CDC indicates that there are 50 or more deaths every day may be due to opiods use. Most common medications related to overdosing and fatal outcomes are narcotic pain-killers like oxycodone (OxyContin), oxymorphone (Opana), and hydrocodone (Vicodin).

"To keep the body in good health is a duty... otherwise we shall not be able to keep our mind strong and clear".

Buddha

CDC Director Thomas Frieden, M.D., M.P.H. said that prescription painkiller abuse is killing more people than cocaine and heroin combined. In his statement, he said that "States, health insurers, health care providers and individuals have critical roles to play in the national effort to stop this epidemic of overdoses while we protect patients who need prescriptions to control pain."[3]

The upsurge in the sale and prescription of these medications for nonmedical purposes is the primary reason behind the deaths related to overdosing. It is evident from the figures reported in the National Survey on Drug Use and Health that in 2010 one in 20 or more than 12 million Americans were using painkillers for a non-medical purpose. This fact is well supported by the data received from Drug Enforcement Administration indicating that since 1999 sales of prescription drugs from pharmacies and hospitals have increased by 300 percent, and the trend is upwards with no sign of halting.

This epidemic results after years of neglecting the data, regarding increasing use of prescription drugs year after year, decade after decade. Non-intended use of medical substances has existed since the earliest days of civilization. It is well documented that the Chinese smoked opium over a thousand years ago. Marijuana has been part of the traditional Indian medicine and religious ceremonies for centuries. The history of alcohol and drug abuse can be traced back to the mythological ages. However, things changed for the worse with better understanding of chemistry, and improved agriculture and extraction abilities. One of the earliest epidemics started in the 19th century when we were able to extract and create more powerful drugs like cocaine from the coca leaves. Although society recognizes abuse with such substances like cocaine and heroin, and its associated risks, prescription drugs are sociologically different.

"We never know how far reaching something we may think, say or do today will affect the lives of millions tomorrow".

B. J. Palmer

Today more and more doctors are coming into the limelight for all the wrong reasons like the highly reported case of the death of Michael Jackson, one of the highest profile deaths linked to the abuse of prescription drugs. It is not an isolated incident. Reports of such tragic outcomes are on the rise with each year, and these tragedies are unfortunately the result of medical carelessness and indifference. The situation in which doctors not only prescribe these drugs, but continue to order refills after refills, results in perpetuating a never ending cycle of destruction of the drug prescription standards and protocols the US medical system.

What is worrisome is that the medical community seems to take this situation lightly. The well-known US guitarist Jimi Hendrix left this world in an untimely manner due to a drug used to treat insomnia called Secobarbital, which he took along with alcohol. The pill was given to him by his girlfriend, who was in turn prescribed the drug by a doctor. His death caused colossal resonance, though it is not clear whether it was an accidental death.

To understand why prescription drugs are so dangerous just consider Elvis Presley. He died due to prescription drug abuse in 1977. Not due to one drug; he was on a cocktail of prescription drugs, taking sedatives, painkillers, anxiolytics, and hypnotics. The investigation into his case revealed that he was prescribed a 5000-10,000 pills in a time span of just eight months. When his treating doctor was asked about such over-prescribing, Doctor G. Nichopoulus said that "Presley felt that by getting the pills from a doctor, he was not a common abuser that got his drugs off the street."

"To enjoy the glow of good health, you must exercise".

Gene Tunney

Such tragic deaths due to the inappropriate prescription of drugs continued through most of the 20th century and only increased in number in the 21st century. Margaux Hemingway died of a fatal dose of phenobarbital, a drug long known for its toxicity. 1999 saw the untimely demise of Dano Plato, due to overduse of muscle relaxants with a painkiller called Vicodin. It is surprising to see how the people continue to abuse prescription drugs.

One of the most prominent and controversial cases that came to attention was the death of Anna Nicole Smith. The reason that this case received national attention is not only due to her tragic drug related death but also because of the fact that just five months before, her son died due to similar circumstances. She died due to a fatal combination of eleven drugs, which were systematically provided to her by her doctor. In fact, there is substantial evidence that her doctor intentionally continued to provide Smith with the drugs. It is a case that highlights the risks, and showcases how doctors can often legally circumvent the law[4].

When it comes to the drug companies, they are easily able to escape from liability by stating that they produce these drugs according to approved standards, and they only sell drugs within the legal framework. Drug manufacturers say that they have nothing to do with the false or over prescriptions by the doctors. While doctors are also not ready to take the blame, they say that they have to prescribe the medications as patients continue to demand them, and thus they are doing their job. In fact, regulatory authorities are already calling it a "catch 22" like situation. Worst of all, everyone seems to be able to claim righteousness for their actions.

"Good health and good sense are two of life's greatest blessings".

Publilius Syrus

The medical community, doctors, researchers, and regulatory bodies each have their own version of the story. They say that each year more than 116 million Americans complain about chronic pain. Though the medical community is supposed to practicing cautiously, it cannot neglect the sheer amount of complaints. Moreover, they must believe that the majority of these complains are true. They have to manage the problem and help the patients. They have to prescribe more and more analgesics both opioid and non-opioid.

All the data leave no doubt that the US is going through the worst epidemic of drug addiction in history, and the worrying part is the change in the pattern of this addiction with the dominance of legal prescription drugs in place of street drugs. It is evident from the analysis of statistics. If we look at the younger age groups, addiction is both due to prescription drugs and recreational drugs sold on the streets. However, addiction is widespread in the elderly populationas well, something new for Americans. There are people who were prescribed opioid painkillers for medical conditions, and then got addicted to them. Most of such people are between the age of 40 to 80, and a large number of them are suffering overdose each year.

Even in young population, many get addicted due to medical reasons. Many young people are prescribed the opioid-based drugs for medical conditions, and they get accustomed to taking them regularly. However, after time, either they are refused or are not provided with enough dosage. No one wants to prescribe healthy looking adults for too long. Thus, they turn towards the street drugs. Many of them start by procuring medical drugs from the black market, however, it is a costly option and these young people soon find it difficult to continue. Then many of them decide to give cheaper heroin a try, resulting in worsening of their addiction.

> "There's nothing more important than our good health - that's our principal capital asset".
>
> **Arlen Specter**

There is no doubt the pharmaceutical industry, researchers, and even doctors are good at data manipulation. The medical community is a big player in this epidemic, yet with the help of statistics and data, they are continuing to hide their role, continuing to hide the fact that these drugs do more harm than good. Admittedly, we would like to think that researchers, regulatory bodies, pharmaceutical companies, doctors, all of them are doing their job with utmost honesty, but this is not always the case as the dollar sings it's siren song.

Consider a report published in the United Kingdom, the story was part of the reporting by The Guardian. They compared extensive data from the trials and found out that trials that were funded by pharmaceutical companies or other industries were more likely to report positive reports, as compared to those independently funded (not supported by pharmaceutical industry). There was a massive outcry at this report with researchers claiming that it is due to the fact that industry endorses research only when they expect positive results. While some went on to explain that they do not have a choice due to a deficit of public funding in scientific research[5]. But whatever the stakeholders say, one thing is quite evident - that most research is industry-funded and biased.

Such reports of biased research and altered data are not just coming from the newspaper. Many articles related to the subject has been published in the more prestigious medical journals. *The BMJ* reported that the industry regularly funds even the most prestigious research bodies and agencies. Therefore the journal found out that the industry on average may pay a consultancy fee to researcher from anywhere between $330,000 to $380000 per annum[6]. That was the consultation fee to researchers in the field of nutrition. Researchers involved in the area of opioids may get much higher fees.

"Medicine is the study of disease and what causes man to die. Chiropractic is the study of health and what causes man to live".

B. J. Palmer

This is not to suggest that drug companies are blatantly manipulating research data. The industry understands that this could have grave consequences. Therefore, to this extent, they can be trusted. Rather they are using the more straightforward strategy of manipulateing the results. They merely discard the negative research, or may not report it at all. If all that is not possible, they will downplay the negative side and continue to focus on and exaggerate the positive results. In that way, it looks as if benefits far outweigh the risks involved with any particular kind of chemotherapy.

Let's clarify one of the most commonly deployed techniques by drug companies. Let's say that a pharmaceutical company has come up with some new molecule and it wants to prove the safety and efficacy of that drug. For this purpose, it starts a clinical trial at ten different sites, and in the trial four sites report negative results, another four report more or less acceptable and positive results, and two sites report something in between. What the company will then do is they will simply disqualify the four sites reporting the negative data, reasons could be any from poor compliance of the participants, to the failure of research sites to meet the pre-set standards. Now the company is left with data that looks positive and more or less realistic. Now they have positive data from four sites where people may have got well for a myriad of differing reasons, rather than necessarily due to the drug being tested. But once the objectives of the pharmaceutical company have been achieved, why bother to go into detail. Thus, everything has been done more or less in a legal way, without visible data manipulation. You the reader would never get to know the truth, and you would only be led to believe that the results were mostly positive.

"The foundation of success in life is good health: that is the substratum fortune; it is also the basis of happiness. A person cannot accumulate a fortune very well when he is sick".

P. T. Barnum

There is no scarcity of stories being published on the subject, though they too often go unnoticed. In 2007, most major newspapers circulated a story about how the pharmaceutical giant Pfizer (one of the largest pharmaceutical companies in the world) manipulated the research data, to show the higher effectiveness of its drug Neurontin in the treatment of disorders other than epilepsy for which it was approved. They were found to be involved in spinning the negative data, to show the drug in better light[7].

Just to prove this point, have a look at the report published by a prestigious of publication: *JAMA*, which is the Journal of the American Medical Association. The journal found that though almost one out of every three elderly adults is on an antidepressant or other similar drug with psychoactive properties, their meta-analysis of all the major clinical trials published between the year 1980 and 2009 did not show that these medicines helped in most cases. Analysis by JAMA clearly states that these drugs, used to correct depression-like state, would only help in severe cases. They found no proof of effectiveness in mild to moderate cases[8].

Industry stakeholders often give the benefit of the doubt in interpreting the research data. Even the best trained medical specialists find it hard to understand data from clinical investigations. This is not to suggest that opioids should not be used at all, or they do not help at all. There is substantial evidence that they do help in moderate to severe pain syndromes, however most of the data published by the pharmaceutical industry are regarding the short-term use of opioid in acute pain relief. Evidence in favor of long-term use are at best, meager. There is a complete absence of long-term publicly funded trials supporting this[9].

"Good health is not something we can buy. However, it can be an extremely valuable savings account".

Anne Wilson Schaef

Much research has been published questioning the long-term use of opioids for various medical conditions. Such opinions though, are often suppressed by the much stronger voice coming from the industry. As the white and Kehlen wrote in their article published in the prestigious journal "we are jumping from frypan into the fire," meaning that overtreatment with opioids is emerging as a colossal challenge[10].

In this game, doctors are pointing fingers at the pharmaceutical companies for providing inaccurate information and data manipulation, as pharmaceutical companies are blaming the doctors for over-prescription of these drugs. While both parties are blaming each other, the epidemic of opioid related mortality continues to rise. The question of who is to be blamed remains unanswered in this whole process.

It seems that in this issue all the three parties involved have their share of responsibility. With individuals feigning symptoms for the sake of obtaining prescriptions and drug manufacturers continuing to manipulate the data, and doctors also continueing to misuse their authority, by either intentionally or unintentionally over-treating pain related conditions with opioids.

The whole epidemic of prescription drugs has been caused by to a combination of factors. These factors could be well summarized as:

- The misconception that if doctors are prescribing it, then it must be good, or at least harmless, especially if compared to the street drugs. However, this is not the case. Opioids and similar drugs are from the same group as the street drugs, they are just slightly altered molecules, with better-improved safety profile in the doses approved. Further, most of those drugs are not well studied for long-term consequences on health.

26

"Treasure the love you receive above all. It will survive long after your good health has vanished".

Og Mandino

- The second important factor is the higher availability of these compounds. Data shows that the prescription of psychoactive drugs rose from 5 million to 45 million from 1991 to 2010, while the prescription of opioid analgesics rose from 75.5 million to 209.5 in the same period. This increase is much higher when compared to the rise in population or incidence of disease.

- Finally, people cite various reasons for abuse, which could be explained by the higher prevalence of depression, anxiety, caused by the modern lifestyle. Prolonged lifespan means that people suffer more from chronicl diseases, pain and such. They often find refuge in drug abuse.

To resolve this problem, all the stakeholders must accept their responsibility. Doctors should follow the guidelines more strictly, without obliging patients. This does not mean to under prescribe analgesics or psychoactive agents, it just means that precautions should be taken, and the risks need to be better understood. At the same time, individuals should also realize that opioids are no solution to their life problems, they are just as toxic as street drugs when taken in the wrong dose, however, all their benefit is lost in their abuse. Of course the producers of prescription drugs must understand their responsibility towards society at large, and stop deferring blame.

Last, but not the least, comes the duty of regulatory bodies. We have not discussed much about their role in the whole epidemic, but again this does not mean that they have less relevance.

"While other professions are concerned with changing the environment to suit the weakened body, chiropractic is concerned with strengthening the body to suit the environment".

B. J. Palmer

Much depends on how well the FDA understands the problem. It is, after all, the apex body which controls the functioning of the pharmaceutical industry. The FDA has created The Opioid Policy Steering Committee in May 2017. It has released a statement outlining various steps that the FDA will take to reduce the ensuing epidemic of opioid abuse. The FDA has started implementing significant changes in product packaging and dispensing. How, when, and what changes will be implemented remains to be seen[11].

References

1. CDC. Understanding the Epidemic | Drug Overdose | CDC Injury Center.
    https://www.cdc.gov/drugoverdose/epidemic/index.html.
    Published November 13, 2017. Accessed December 23, 2017.

2. Aldworth J, Colpe LJ, Gfroerer JC, et al. The National Survey on Drug Use and Health Mental Health Surveillance Study: calibration analysis. *Int J Methods Psychiatr Res.* 2010;19(S1):61-87. doi:10.1002/mpr.312.

3. CDC Online Newsroom - Press Release: November 1, 2011.
    https://www.cdc.gov/media/releases/2011/p1101_flu_pain_ki ller_overdose.html. Accessed December 23, 2017.

4. Duke A. New charges filed in investigation of Anna Nicole Smith death - CNN.com.
    http://edition.cnn.com/2009/SHOWBIZ/09/23/anna.nicole. case/index.html. Published September 23, 2009. Accessed December 23, 2017.

"Maintaining good health should be the primary focus of everyone".

Sangram Singh

---

5. Curtis P, correspondent health. Researchers see bias in private-funded studies. *The Guardian.* http://www.theguardian.com/society/2007/jan/09/health.food. Published January 9, 2007. Accessed December 23, 2017.

6. Gornall J. Sugar: spinning a web of influence. *BMJ.* 2015;350:h231. doi:10.1136/bmj.h231.

7. Saul S. Experts Conclude Pfizer Manipulated Studies. *The New York Times.* https://www.nytimes.com/2008/10/08/health/research/08drug.html. Published October 8, 2008. Accessed December 23, 2017.

8. Fournier JC, DeRubeis RJ, Hollon SD, et al. Antidepressant Drug Effects and Depression Severity: A Patient-Level Meta-analysis. *JAMA.* 2010;303(1):47-53. doi:10.1001/jama.2009.1943.

9. Rosenblum A, Marsch LA, Joseph H, Portenoy RK. Opioids and the Treatment of Chronic Pain: Controversies, Current Status, and Future Directions. *Exp Clin Psychopharmacol.* 2008;16(5):405-416. doi:10.1037/a0013628.

32

"Health is the greatest gift, contentment the greatest
wealth, faithfulness the best relationship."

Buddha

---

10. White PF, Kehlet H. Improving Pain Management: Are We Jumping from the Frying Pan into the Fire? *Anesth Analg.* 2007;105(1):10-12. doi:10.1213/01.ane.0000268392.05157.a8.

11. Commissioner FDA. Press Announcements - Statement from FDA Commissioner Scott Gottlieb, M.D., on new strategies for addressing the crisis of opioid addiction through innovation in packaging, storage and disposal. https://www.fda.gov/NewsEvents/Newsroom/PressAnnouncements/ucm582954.htm. Published October 30, 2017. Accessed December 23, 2017.

"A healthy attitude is contagious but don't wait to catch it from others." Be a carrier.

Tom Stoppard

Chapter 2

Navigating through the current health care system

The United States health care system is currently a mix of government programs, private enterprise capitalism, and government agencies that oversee and regulate the various aspects of State and Federal programs as well as private enterprise. Many people feel that our current system is "broken" and inadequate. The Affordable Health Care Act, sometimes called Obamacare, was an attempt to Federalize all of health care in America and incorporate all of it under one clearing house. The recent repeal of the "mandate", a law requiring private citizens to purchase private health care insurance which met certain criteria established by the government, has largely taken the teeth out of the governments ability to control the private sector and determine what types of care are available and required. Recently, Insurance companies have begun to offer policies which do not cover all of the services and procedures which the government had previously mandated that everyone should carry. This will affect the private market in many ways. Government programs are still very closely controlled by their respective governing parties and the insurance companies which underwrite them where applicable. The Federal Government is in charge of the care of military veterans, and some federal employees, under the Veterans Administration. This is a pseudo single payer system which provides care to those eligible to varying degrees in accordance with their history of Federal or Military Service. There are many benefits to the VA healthcare system, as well as many problems, which is not surprising in a large government bureaucracy.

"The master maker of the human body did not create you and then run off and leave you masterless. He stayed on the job as innate, as the fellow within, as nerve transmission controlling every function of life, as spirit from above-down, inside-out, expressing, creating, exploring, directing you in every field and phase of experience so that your home is truly the world and the world is your home".

B. J. Palmer

The VA operates independently and in conjunction with other health care outlets. Navigating the VA could be, and is in fact, the subject of entire books and will not be addressed here specifically. Medicaid is a state program in each of the various states and is mandated and controlled by the federal government. Worker's Compensation is also a state level program mandated and controlled by the federal government, and underwritten, in most cases, by private insurance companies. Medicare is a Federal program originally designed to take care of the elderly and certain other classes of people who don't have access to care that they would need. Medicare was the result of previous attempts to institute a national single payer health care system for all Americans. This could not get passed through several administrations, from President Truman in 1945, through John F Kennedy, and a compromise to cover seniors in 1965 under Lyndon B. Johnson was finally passed. In 1972 president Nixon expanded Medicare to cover people with long-term disabilities and those with end stage renal disease. In the early 2000's people with ALS (Lou Gehrig's disease) were added to the roles. Medicare has a Part A which covers hospital insurance and Part B which covers regular doctor visits. In the private insurance sector, many insurance companies employ or emulate Medicare standards. Many Medicare laws and restrictions govern care outside of the Medicare realm, such as pricing.

With this big mish-mash of systems and programs, complicated by the interests of large pharmaceutical companies and the interests of the insurance companies, it can be very difficult to navigate your way through our current health care system while ensuring that your health is the number one priority.

"Ill-health of body or of mind, is defeat. Health alone is victory. Let all men, if they can manage it, contrive to be healthy!"

Thomas Carlyle

At the writing of this book, The World Health Organization (WHO) ranks the United States as number 37 in a world ranking of health care systems. American health care is recognized as the worst of the worlds 12 richest nations. The health of Americans is the worst of the top 16 developed countries. America has higher rate of adverse birth outcomes, injuries and homicide, adolescent pregnancy, STD's, Drug use, obesity and diabetes, heart disease, chronic lung disease, disabilities and arthritis. Many of these may be the result of political and social factors or education, others are clearly a result of poor health care directly. Italy, Iceland and Switzerland are ranked as the 3 healthiest countries in the world. The United States ranks number 19 in high BMI (Body Mass Index) worldwide, but number 1 in developed countries. The United States spends far more on health care than other countries, by far. At over $8,000 per person annually, we pass Norway, the 2nd highest by more than $2,000 per year, and almost double the average rate of developed countries. One would expect Americans to be the healthiest people in the world, but they are not. Let's explore some of the reasons why this may be, and how you can get the most health out of your dollar.

Let's begin by examining some of the problems with our health care system. Some issues, such as the cost of healthcare under federal and state programs, will not be under the control of the healthcare consumer. Others will. To begin our exploration, we should examine some of the reasons behind the high cost of healthcare. We have already identified that government run healthcare costs, along with their huge administrative bureaucracies, will not be something that the individual consumer can effect; which is not to imply that the public at large cannot address the issue and hold our representatives more responsible to control these costs. Many people believe that tort reform (civil liability court action such as malpractice) will reduce healthcare costs.

"The best six doctors anywhere and no one can deny it are sunshine, water, rest, air, exercise and diet."

Wayne Fields

This has become a political issue in the United States, as do most important issues, with reasonable arguments on both sides. In fact, it is possible that carefully crafted tort reform could reduce healthcare costs to some degree. Studies suggest that caps on malpractice awards and other such actions could aggregately shave as much as 5% off the end cost of premiums for the consumer. The cost of malpractice insurance can be very high. An Obstetrician may pay as much as $200,000 per year for coverage, which of course, translates to higher costs on the consumer end. On the other hand, Chiropractors pay an average of $500 per year, which does not translate to savings because the prices for Chiropractic care are mandated by the Medicare administration. So, as you can see, this subject is complicated. United States citizens do not use more healthcare than other countries, so why does it cost so much more? In fact, it has been demonstrated that healthcare is more expensive in the United States than other countries. There are many reasons for this. Some argue that under single payer systems (Socialized Medicine), which many European countries have, the government is able to negotiate better prices than insurance companies in the United States do. I have my personal doubts about the efficacy of using politicians in negotiations, but this is one argument. In fact, Canada does have lower prices on pharmaceuticals, but it isn't because of the negotiating prowess of Canadian politicians and bureaucrats, it's because the patent laws of the United States artificially prop up the prices of new drugs on the U.S. Market so that the pharmaceutical companies can make a profit. Before you condemn them for this, remember that without a profit motive these new drugs would not be developed or marketed; so no profit equals no pharmaceutical development. Other reasons for higher costs are the complications of diabetes in United States healthcare because of our high rate of obesity. Obesity is actually a large driver of healthcare costs in the United States, and that cost is diffused over the entire industry.

42

"There's nothing more important than our good health –

that's our principal capital asset."

Arlen

Another big driver of high healthcare costs is the delivery systems we have in America. Because so many people don't have healthcare insurance, or have government subsidized health insurance, they use hospitals and emergency rooms as portal of entry for their issues. This means that since hospitals cannot turn people away legally, people without coverage or money can receive care if they go to a hospital rather than to a regular family doctor's office. For many people on government healthcare plans the same rules apply. Hospital admittance is much more expensive than regular doctors offices because of numerous regulations governing hospital admittance and what services are required and available at that portal. These costs must be absorbed into the portion of the population which pays for healthcare as hospitals, like other businesses, cannot afford to operate if they give their services out for free. This is why hospital costs are so inflated. Another reason related to this is that pricing schedules are mandated by insurance companies, and some services may be covered, even if they're not the best option, while others are not. A good example is mammography. It is an old, outdated procedure which is not very good comparatively at detecting early breast cancer. Thermography is much more effective in general, but is not covered. It's also much cheaper. But mammography is covered, and the machines are very expensive, so everyone pays more, and gets less, because the machines have to be payed for, and thermography isn't covered. I have seen in practice that for many people, the covered procedure is the preferred procedure, even when it's not the best procedure. I have seen many people get back surgery that they didn't need, and didn't do well with, because decompression therapy isn't covered, but surgery is, and it costs much more. The American public regards paying cash for healthcare as anathema in general. They are accustomed to health insurance, and they are trusting of the insurance companies to make the choices that are in their best interests.

"The power that made the body, HEALS THE BODY. It happens no other way".

B. J. Palmer

There are other approaches to healthcare. So far we have discussed the institutions and the general model of healthcare which has been developed to serve the medical, or allopathic model of healthcare which is designed to address healthcare concerns as issues arise. When you develop a problem, you go to the doctor. The doctor addresses the issue, usually with a drug, sometimes with a surgery, and sometimes by some other means. The insurance company pays the bill, hopefully, and you go on your way. There are many differentiation s in modern healthcare, and many specialists. You may have a GP (general practitioner) who is your first line doctor. If your problem is more complicated he may send you to a specialist. There are many different specialties including Obstetrics, Pediatricians for children, Gynecologists for women's specific issues, Oncologists for cancer, Podiatrists for your feet. Orthopedists for your joints, Cardiologists for your heart, Phrenologists for your kidneys, ENT's for ears, nose and throat, Internists for your organs, and on and on. There are non-doctor specialists such as Physical Therapists, Phlebotomists, radiologists, Nurse practitioners that can serve as a family doctor or anesthesiologist, PA's or Physician Assistants that can also serve essentially as a doctor under the supervision of another doctor. How do you know where to go? Most people just go their primary provider and the get referred to wherever that doctor deems appropriate. Is that always the best way to go? Are you getting sent to the best specialist, or to your doctors buddy from college who needs a little help with his practice? Or someone they met at the last convention? How do you know? Are they just passing you around because you have great insurance and you're a gold mine? Have you had an MRI of the same thing four different times for four different doctors? I've seen these things happen. How do you avoid this and insure that your health is the number one priority? It's so complicated how can anyone be sure?

"The wish for healing has always been half of health."

Lucius Annaeus Seneca

There is a model that I recommend. The first thing you need to do is find a practitioner whom you trust and feel comfortable with. This person will coordinate and manage your health care. It doesn't matter what they are, they could be an MD who practices as a GP, a Nurse Practitioner, a Physician's assistant, a Chiropractor, an Acupuncturist, Homeopath or whatever. Whom you choose should be someone you trust and someone who sees health care similarly to how you do. It is also important that they not be too partisan. Some practitioners are very slanted in how they see health care. Some Medical doctors would never recommend a Chiropractor, even if that's your best option simply because they don't like them. That's not serving your interest, that's serving their ego. There are Physical Therapists who would never recommend a Chiropractor, I even know of one who bans his patients from seeing Chiropractors. There are Chiropractors who would never send you to a Medical doctor, no matter how grievous your condition is. That won't serve your interests either. No matter how good they are, they can't help you with a ruptured appendix. I'm partial to using a Chiropractor as a primary provider, but that's because I am one and I know that a good one will be more concerned with your best interests than with forcing you to accept their philosophy. I believe in Chiropractic philosophy, but I also believe that educating you so that you understand why it's correct is my job, not forcing you to accept it by guilt or misleading you. You need to come to this understanding on your own or it's not going to serve you. Sometimes, two specialties working in conjunction is the best. Chiropractic and Physical Therapy are an excellent example. They almost always both work better when paired. Some health care practitioners want to maintain domain over their patients so that they do not lose them. If you do a good job, you won't lose them. If you try to keep them loyal to yourself when it's not in their best interest, you will eventually lose them for sure.

48

"No matter how much it gets abused, the body can restore balance. The first rule is to stop interfering with nature."

Deepak Chopra

The best thing any practitioner can ever do for their patient is make sure that they are aware of all of their options, know the real pros and cons of each, and make their own choices, because in the end the patient is the one that has to live with the decision. It's good to help and inform the patient, but not to coerce them. Keep all of these things in mind when you choose a primary practitioner. There is a lot of misinformation in the health care field, find someone who will be honest with you, and hopefully not too biased. Health care practitioners are people, and of course to a Surgeon, surgery is your best option. To a lot of MD's, prescriptions are your best option. To an Acupuncturist, Acupuncture can treat almost any condition. I know because I do Acupuncture as well. A good primary practitioner is going to manage all of your health care. They are going to need to know everything you are doing in your healthcare. They need to know all of your prescriptions. They need to know all of the specialists you are going to. They need to know everything in your health history, not just the things that you think pertain to their specialty. They can't manage your whole health care panoply unless they know everything in it. I get so many patients who leave things out because they think I don't need to know. I need to know every surgery you've had. I need to know if you are on blood thinners if I'm going to do acupuncture on you. I need to know if you have osteoporosis if I'm going to adjust your rib that's out of place. I don't want to break it. I see people all the time who give me prescription lists with redundant prescriptions because they have one doctor putting them on one thing, and another doctor putting them on another drug that does the exact same thing; neither doctor knows that they're taking both. Your primary care provider needs to be able to manage all of this. If you take a lot of prescriptions, I recommend that you choose a Medical doctor to do this and not a Chiropractor or Homeopath who may not be as familiar with all of the new drugs that keep coming out.

"To keep the body in good health is a duty… otherwise, we shall not be able to keep our mind strong and clear."

Buddha

If you're someone who is averse to surgery or taking pills, I would recommend you not use a Medical doctor as primary. Choose someone who reflects the way you approach healthcare, because that's what you're going to get in the end.

So you may think to yourself that you've never really considered this, and you don't know where to start. The approach I recommend is pretty simple. I recommend that you approach treatment from the perspective of least invasive to most invasive. Least invasive includes things that aren't extreme measures first, and most invasive is doing the most extreme treatments. Good examples of least invasive treatments are changing your diet and exercise in response to healthcare issues. Most invasive would be going straight to surgery for any issue that comes up such as getting a nerve ablation (burning your nerves out) for a pain. There are usually many appropriate steps in between. In my view, a general listing of least to most invasive would be diet and exercise as a first step, followed by Chiropractic care and/or Physical Therapy and/or massage therapy, followed by pharmaceutical intervention, followed by surgery as usually a last resort. There is a difference between curative care and palliative care. Curative care seeks to end the condition that causes the symptom. Palliative care seeks to lessen or eliminate the symptoms, but does not treat the underlying condition. Some people only seek curative care, some people only care about palliative care. I am not here to judge which you should choose, they both have their place. In my model of ideal healthcare, I put the emphasis on curative care and resort to palliative care as a last resort, when the underlying problem cannot be resolved such as in type I diabetes. I see patients seeking both types of care, and I gladly provide both. For example, there are people who are very overweight, work at a desk or drive a truck, and have a lot of lower back pain. They need to exercise and lose weight, but some of them don't want to or it isn't a high enough priority.

52

"Many of us take better care of our automobiles than we do our own bodies... yet the auto has replaceable parts".

B. J. Palmer

I don't turn them away, I treat them. Repeatedly. That's OK. I educate them as best I can, and then I let them decide. It's not my life, it's not my decision. Many times I see people who are misled. They have been convinced that they need a surgery that they don't need. They come to me as a last resort. They got lucky, because I've also seen a lot of unnecessary surgeries after it's too late, and I can't fix that. It's too late. Always get a second opinion before non-emergency surgery. The goal of healthcare, in my opinion, is to approach homeostasis as closely as possible. Homeostasis is the condition where everything in your body is working correctly and in concert in perfect harmony. I say as closely as possible because most of us cannot reach 100% homeostasis. If you've had an organ removed, you can't be 100% because that organ had a purpose, and your body no longer does that. If you take a prescription, you can't be 100% because that drug affects your metabolism in a thousand ways, known and unknown, so that your body isn't working exactly as designed. You can, however, approach homeostasis as closely as your own body will allow. That, to me, is the goal of healthcare. Some people think that the goal of healthcare is to be symptom free. These are not the same thing. Your body is very adept at compensation and will adjust to varying conditions to adapt itself and run as best as possible, and symptoms only appear when your body reaches it's limit and can't compensate anymore. Painkillers are an example of a treatment that stretches the ability of the body to not have symptoms by shutting down the signals that your body is sending to tell you that there is a problem. This is a good approach to treating things like RSD (reflex sympathetic dystrophy) which is a condition where the body produces pain for reasons that we don't yet understand fully, and therefore can't treat the cause, or pain from terminal cancer, but it's a terrible approach to treating everyday aches and pains from known, treatable causes. If you're having a handful of Tylenol or Ibuprofen for breakfast everyday, you're not really doing yourself any favors.

"The greatest wealth is health."

Virgil

Some of the common things I see in my office are migraine headaches and sciatica, or leg pains misdiagnosed as sciatica. The normal regimen people seem to follow for migraines is taking pills first. I did. Sometimes this works, more commonly not. Following that, they will go to all sorts of specialists. They may get stronger prescription drugs, sometimes surgery, nerve ablation, or even Botox, which is basically botulinum food poisoning injected int their nerves to kill them so that you can't feel pain anymore, sort of a chemical ablation. At some point, some people will wander into a Chiropractic office, sometimes from a referral, sometimes out of desperation, and discover that there actually is a biomechanical cause to most migraine headaches and Chiropractic will actually rid you of them. You will never know that if you rely on the standard medical model. Sciatica I another problem that people go to extremes to get treated, when, in fact, it's usually a rather simple problem for most Chiropractors to resolve. Sciatica is almost always caused by the sciatic nerve being constricted by an anatomical deviation anywhere from the spinal cord, through the vertebrae, across the sacro-iliac joint, over the piriformis muscle, and down the leg. Your Chiropractor can figure out where with a few simple tests, and usually correct it. The normal route of treatment consists of painkillers for as long as they work. When your body no longer responds to that, we move on to steroid injections, which act as a stronger more direct painkiller. Most people will quickly build a tolerance to that, so then the next step may be an epidural where they inject painkillers directly into your spinal cord to stop the pain signals to your brain (you still hurt,but you don't know it). Next comes surgery. There are two common ones for this. There is the laminectomy, where the back side of your vertebra is removed to let the nerves float around freely, and there's the lumbar fusion, which usually follows scraping the arthritic growths off of the vertebrae to address stenosis, which is a fancy word for "closing up" of a natural hole or passageway in the bone where the nerve goes through.

"I believe that the greatest gift you can give your family

and the world is a healthy you."

Joyce Meyer

The lumbar fusion consists of bolting the vertebrae together with braces and screws so that they can't move anymore. Sometimes this follows a diskectomy, where the vertebral disks are removed if they are bulged or damaged. In most cases, Chiropractic adjustments, and Decompression therapy if there are disk problems, would have fixed the problem years before you even got to this point, and reserved function, hence maintaining homeostasis. Every surgery reduces the the degree to which you can enjoy complete health permanently. Sometimes it's necessary, most often not. Another common problem I see is GERD, or reflux, which is usually first treated with acid reducing pills, and then eventually with a cholecystectomy, or gallbladder surgery. In most cases this problem stems from a transitory hiatal hernia, where the lack of muscle tone, or excess weight, causes the top of the stomach to protrude through the diaphragm, pinching it off beneath the cardiac sphincter, which is the muscle ring that closes the stomach, keeping the stomach from closing at the esophagus. This allows acid up into the esophagus with pain from the acis erosion which ensues. When it's due to muscle flaccidity and not excess weight, it's normally because the superior mesanteric nerve is pinched off where it exits the spinal cord at the T4, T5, and T6 vertebrae and the "close" signal to the stomach can't get through and the internal abdominal muscles don't keep the stomach in place. You're supposed to have a gallbladder. Do you really want to lose it when there's a simple adjustment that can fix the problem without giving up your internal organs? Most people enjoy diarrhea for the rest of their lives after losing their gallbladder because they can no longer digest fats. While you're in the first stages and still taking the little purple pills, you will lose the ability to digest protein at least to some degree as that I one purpose of your stomach acid. Another purpose of stomach acid, which acid reflux pills defeat, is that it purges contaminants and infectious bacteria from your gut. Your stomach is supposed to be acid.

"Cheerfulness is the best promoter of health and is as friendly to the mind as to the body."

Joseph Addison

There are innumerable conditions that I see over treated every day that could have been treated with Chiropractic or physical therapy, but went to surgery, or got strung out so long on prescription medications which suppressed the symptoms, that they had to go to surgery because the level of degradation was so great. Osteoarthritis is the perfect example. Osteoarthritis is wear and tear on your joints from misalignment. Everyone has it. Nobody needs to. It is completely preventable in theory. Healthy movement with aligned joints prevents it. Most people get a joint out of alignment and the first treatment is pills. That make the pain go away, but the grinding keeps on, quietly in the background, until it gets adjusted - if it gets adjusted. If not, the joint degrades and osteoarthritis is the product. Osteoarthritis is not a disease, it's a result. Rheumatoid arthritis is a disease.

So where do I go from here? You've found a practitioner. They match your outlook on healthcare. They're competent in the issues that you have. You've decided whether curative or palliative care is more important to you, and your provider is someone who will respect your views. Now I would take an inventory of my own various health concerns and determine if I'm addressing them in the best manner in line with my views. I would determine if the healthcare providers I am seeing are the best ones for me. I would consider if there was more I could be doing for my own health. Most health problems that people suffer are the result of lifestyle habits. Is there anything I need to start doing or stop doing? Is there more I need to learn about my specific issues. Have I been blindly trusting the advice of people in the field? You wouldn't blindly trust the car salesman to make your choices for you, why would you trust anyone else with their inherent biases and priorities to make your healthcare choices? We live in the world of free information. You don't need to learn everything, but learn enough to ask good questions.

"The preservation of health is easier than the cure for

disease".

B. J. Palmer

In other chapters we have addressed the use of drugs, the benefits of chiropractic care, some common misconceptions in healthcare, and other subjects which could easily be elaborated more in this chapter. Without being redundant, I will generally review a few of the basic concepts which I think are really relevant here.

We get one body. We want it to last as long as possible and be in good running condition. The human body is inherently wise and knows how to operate correctly. I Chiropractic we call this "innate". It refers to the innate wisdom of the body to operate in it's environment and adapt to changes and respond. It also refers to the innate "intelligence" of the universe which abides by the laws of physics and is responsible for the functioning of all that is. It is inherent in everything. It is inherent in you. It is wiser than the collective knowledge of man, and it can create and maintain life. When your body is working perfectly it is in a state of homeostasis. Homeostasis is the ideal state of physiological being and is in harmony with innate. It is the goal of innate. Throughout life we collect bumps and bruises and misalignments and asymmetries and damage that interfere with homeostasis. It can't be avoided, it's the process of living, it's why we are temporary and get replaced by new generations. Healthcare is ideally the means by which we maintain our homeostasis as well as we can for as long as we can so that we can be alive and healthy as long as possible. Curative care is core to this. Palliative care is core to comfort and not necessarily a contributing factor to health, and in fact is often a detriment to homeostasis. Products and procedures which contribute to homeostasis are preferable to those which degrade it. Exercise is good, our bodies are designed to move and work and they break down and degrade without it. Good food is essential to fueling our bodies. Drugs are not good for your body in most cases. All medications are poisons metered out in dosages which have desireable side effects. They also have negative side effects. Allopathy (traditional medicine) is the art of balancing the application of medicine.

62

> "To get rich never your risk your health. For it is the truth that health is the wealth of wealth."
>
> **Richard Baker**

Ideally, homeostasis requires no medication. Surgery is a last resort as it permanently degrades or alters the natural design of the body. Sometimes it is necessary. Almost all non-emergency surgery can be avoided. A post surgical body can never enjoy 100% homeostasis. A medicated body can never enjoy 100% homeostasis. Most wear and tear of life precludes 100% homeostasis. There are many different models of healthcare available in the United States. Most healthcare decisions are subjective, no matter what anyone tells you. Healthcare professionals are salesmen the same as any other profession, and like a carpenter with a hammer only sees nails, they see what their specialty is your health concerns. No one will ever accept responsibility for your healthcare outcomes to a higher degree than you will. You have a responsibility to yourself to get second opinions, to have a central healthcare "manager" who knows all your issues and treatments, and to seek care that coincides with your view of healthcare as ultimately you will be the person who has to live with the decisions that either you have made, or have allowed someone else to make for you. Least invasive care is preferable to most invasive care because it degrades the degree to which you can achieve homeostasis the least. Less invasive care never precludes more invasive care as an option in the event that it doesn't work. More invasive care often precludes less invasive care and if it doesn't work you will lose those options. I can't tell you how many times I've seen people who've had a surgery with a poor outcome for a problem that I probably could have treated successfully, but now I can't. I can't adjust a low back after its been fused. I can't adjust a lunate bone in the wrist to alleviate carpal tunnel syndrome after the flexor retinaculum has been destroyed by carpal tunnel surgery. It's too late. If you tried the adjustment first and it didn't work, you could still get the surgery, but the reverse is not true. I cannot alleviate the pain of arthritis after ten years of Ibuprofen have allowed it to degrade to stage 3 or stage 4 arthrosis. Choose wisely, you can't go to a showroom and pick out a new body after this one is used up. Not yet.

"You are not your illness. You have an individual story to tell. You have a name, a history, a personality. Staying yourself is part of the battle."

Julian Seifte

CHAPTER 3

THE GERM THEORY IS A MYTH

Why Is The Germ Theory Controversial?

Germs are everywhere. The "germ theory" that people use to explain disease, is a carry-over from the early 1800s. These microscopic organisms are one of the most misunderstood factors of health. Like plant seeds, germs need the proper environment to become recognizable diseases. The viruses and bacteria that we call germs are everywhere. They're in food, air, water and all over us. However, germs no more cause disease than cars cause automobile accidents. When our bodies provide a hospitable environment for germs to flourish, they can cause disease.

Germ theory denialism is the belief that germs do not cause infectious disease, and that the germ theory of disease is wrong. It usually involves arguing that Louis Pasteur's model of infectious disease was wrong and that Antoine Béchamp's was right. One of the first movements to deny the germ theory was the Sanitary Movement, which was nevertheless central in developing America's public health infrastructure. One well-known advocate of this form of denialism is Bill Maher, who has claimed that Pasteur recanted germ theory on his deathbed. Shikha Dalmia, writing in The Washington Examiner, referred to Maher as a "germ theory denier" after he made these comments on Real Time with Bill Maher on March 4, 2007. However, in response to criticism of his views, Maher said, on the October 16, 2009 episode of his show, that he accepted microorganisms as the cause of some disease, but expressed skepticism about other topics in medicine, such as vaccination.

"Rest when you're weary. Refresh and renew yourself, your body, your mind, your spirit. Then get back to work."

Ralph Marston

Similarly, the following month, Maher wrote that he "understand germ theory," but that he still thought that "Western medicine ignores the fact that the terrain in which bacteria can thrive is crucial and often controllable, which shouldn't even be controversial.

Who was Louis Pasteur?

Louis Pasteur was born in Dole, Eastern France. He was a conscientious and hard-working student, though not considered exceptional. One of his professors called him 'mediocre'. He received a doctorate in 1847, and after obtaining posts at Strasbourg, Lille, and Paris, he spent much time researching aspects of Chemistry. One key discovery of his was in research on tartrate acid showing the crystals contained a mirror image of right-handed and left-handed isomers.

His most important discoveries were in the field of germ study. He showed that germs required certain micro-organisms to develop; using this knowledge, he found that the fermentation of yeast could be delayed. Louis Pasteur then turned to practical ways of killing bacteria in liquids such as milk. His process of pasteurization successfully killed bacteria in milk without destroying milk protein. This was a radical discovery and made drinking milk safer. The process of pasteurization was named after him, and it saved many lives.

Louis Pasteur was a great believer in hard work, never content to rest on his laurels, he continued to work very hard in his laboratory to develop more cures. In 1860 the French Academy announced a prize of 2,500 Francs to anyone who provided convincing experimental proof for or against the spontaneous generation theory of life.

Pasteur was awarded the prize in 1862. He showed that no microbes ever grew in nutrient solutions which had been sterilized by heating, provided the air above the solutions was also sterilized.

"So what Chiropractic does, is that it simply "takes the handcuffs off Nature", as it were. By finding the particular vertebra that had shifted and restoring it to its natural position, the adjustment thus releases the natural flow of nerve impulse. When the maze of nerves, or Nature's communication system, supplies the body with the energy it needs for well-being, you have health".

B. J. Palmer

If unsterilized air was allowed into space above the solutions, microbes began growing in the solutions. The microbes were present in the unheated air.

The Pasteur Institute was opened in 1888. During Louis Pasteur's lifetime, it was not easy for him to convince others of his ideas, controversial in their time but considered absolutely correct today. Pasteur fought to convince surgeons that germs existed and carried diseases, and dirty instruments and hands spread germs and therefore disease. Pasteur's pasteurization process killed germs and prevented the spread of disease.

Louis Pasteur had great faith in the good nature of humans. He worked tirelessly to deliver real benefits for the treatment of infectious diseases. More than any other person, Louis Pasteur helped to increase average life expectancy in the late nineteenth and early twentieth Century.

Achievements of Louis Pasteur

- Process of Pasteurisation making milk safe to drink

- Cure for Rabies

- Cure for anthrax

- His principles were used by later scientists such as Frankland, Valley Radot, Emile Duclaux, Descours and Holmes in developing vaccines for diseases such as typhus, diphtheria, cholera, yellow fever and different strains of plague.

How Did He Discover The Germ Theory?

Proving the germ theory of disease was the crowning achievement of the French scientist Louis Pasteur.

"To insure good health: Eat lightly, breathe deeply, live moderately, cultivate cheerfulness, and maintain an interest in life."

William Londen

He was not the first to propose that diseases were caused by microscopic organisms, but the view was controversial in the 19th century, and opposed the accepted theory of "spontaneous generation".

Pasteur set out to understand the fermentation process, and soon realized that alcohol in wine was produced by yeast which lived on the skins of grapes. During fermentation, the yeast appeared healthy and budding under a microscope, but lactic acid was formed and the wine turned to vinegar when other microbes were seen among the yeast cells. Further analysis of the wine showed a number of complex organic molecules, some of which were able to rotate light, a property of compounds produced by living organisms. Through several experiments, Pasteur showed that fermentation required contact with dust in the air.

Pasteur then turned his attention to the health of silkworms, which produced silk for the cloth industry. He discovered that he found that healthy silk-worms became ill when they nested in the bedding of those suffering from the disease. In this study, Pasteur found that environment directly affected contagion and that the spread of disease could be controlled by sterilization. His studies on yeast had shown that microbes could be airborne, and he realized that these two studies could be directly applied to the transmission of disease in humans.

The final proof of germ theory came when Pasteur was able to grow the anthrax bacillus in culture. Although anthrax had been isolated by Robert Koch, opponents believed that the spores he found could have been containments in his culture medium. Pasteur placed a drop of blood from a sheep dying of anthrax into a sterile culture and allowed the bacilli to grow. He repeated this process until none of the original cultures remained in the final dish. The final culture produced anthrax when injected into sheep, showing that the bacillus was responsible for the disease.

"The natural healing force in each one of us is the greatest force in getting well."

Hippocrates

Why Is It Considered To Not Be Correct?

According to Louis Pasteur's widely accepted germ theory, many illnesses are caused by these micro-organisms and we must protect ourselves and our children from them. Conversely, the human bowel could not function without digestive bacteria, so it isn't necessarily that simple.

Let us re-visit the germ theory. If we are at the mercy of these little foes called bacteria and viruses in our environment, then why aren't we all affected? Have you ever wondered why a group of people exposed to an equal measure of the same germs, respond differently? Take the recent swine flu for instance, why did some die, some got sick and got better, and others were unaffected? If we were truly at the mercy of this virus, wouldn't we all be dead? This may sound a little extreme, but why are some affected and others untouched? Is it bad luck? Is it a sheer chance? Or are there other factors at play here?

Germs are generally opportunistic. This means that they can only "attack" if given the proper opportunity. The opportunity meaning, of course, a weak host, or person with a weakened immune system. If your immune system is weak you can become a target, you are now an opportunity. This can easily be seen in the increased susceptibility of the elderly, the very young, or in cases such as people with AIDS. For example, an Aids patient can simply die from the common cold due to the decreased function of the immune system. So are germs really the culprit? Are we victims of germs? Or are we victims of a weakened immune system?

Why Is The Environment Considered To Be More Important Than The Germ?

74

"A healthy outside starts from the inside."

Robert Urich

The germ theory of disease is based on the concept that many diseases are caused by infections with microorganisms, typically only visualized under high magnification. Such microorganisms can consist of bacterial, viral, fungal, or protist species. Although the growth and productive replication of microorganisms are the cause of disease, environmental and genetic factors may predispose a host or influence the severity of the infection. For example, in a host that is immune-compromised (e.g., due to AIDS or old age), an infection may result in more severe outcomes than in individuals who are fully immunocompetent.

In 1876, Robert Koch was struggling to convince the world that germs cause disease. Today, environmental degradation is a pervasive planetary condition, but the causes remain shrouded in the same popular murk that made diseases mysterious before the work of Koch and Louis Pasteur. For environmental issues, such as the decline of coral reefs, skeptics demand detailed evidence — we must know the exact cause and show that any proposed cures will work.

There is an apocryphal story that Pasteur renounced his germ theory on his death-bed, saying that "Bernard is right. The microbe is nothing. The environment is everything." Germ Theory itself is unsubstantiated even today, but Pasteur himself, in one of the most quoted deathbed statements perhaps of all time, recanted the theory and admitted that he thought his rivals were right and that it was not the germ that caused the disease, but rather the environment in which the germ was found.

What Is The Host Theory?

In host theory, people don't "catch" germs that give them diseases. Instead, disease-causing germs are actually opportunistic, thriving in people whose bodies have a weakness or imbalance internally. They are a byproduct of the disease, not a cause of the disease.

"Smile and smile often. Smile regularly. Smile when you don't feel like it and you will feel like it when you smile".

B. J. Palmer

You see, you have staph, cancer, viruses, and bacteria in you and on you all the time, every day! A healthy balance of beneficial bacteria and healthy body environment keep the unhealthy stuff in balance. If you destroy everything by using antibacterial soaps regularly or using antibiotics every time you feel ill, then you aren't just destroying the bad bacteria, you're also destroying all the beneficial balance too, leaving yourself more susceptible to developing disease.

Unlike Pasteur, who spawned a mentality of fearfully killing germs to prevent disease, Béchamp essentially understood the balance of and the importance of the environment we create with foods that our internal systems can use to either support or not support disease conditions.

Béchamp theorized that germs were benefitted by the chemical byproducts and the degenerative aspects of the unbalanced state of a body. For the disease to take hold there already had to be cellular dysfunction, dead tissue, and other detritus in the body. That's when the germ or bacteria shows and sets up shop because the body or an area of the body is in a state that lets them thrive and gives them a home. This cellular dysfunction or dead tissue can be caused by malnutrition or exposure to toxins, or stress.

Who Discovered The Host Theory? Who Was Antoine Béchamp?

Pierre Jacques Antoine Béchamp (October 16, 1816 – April 15, 1908) was a French scientist now best known for breakthroughs in applied organic chemistry and for a bitter rivalry with Louis Pasteur. He was educated at the University of Strasbourg, receiving a doctor of science degree in 1853 and doctor of medicine in 1856, and ran a pharmacy in the city. In 1854 was appointed Professor of Chemistry at the University of Strasbourg, a post previously held by Louis Pasteur.

"The sovereign invigorator of the body is exercise, and of all the exercises walking is the best."

Thomas Jefferson

Béchamp developed the Béchamp reduction, an inexpensive method to produce aniline dye, permitting Perkin to launch the synthetic-dye industry. Béchamp also synthesized the first organic arsenic drug, arsanilic acid, from which Ehrlich later synthesized the first chemotherapeutic drug. Béchamp's rivalry with Pasteur was initially for priority in attributing fermentation to microorganisms, later for attributing the silkworm disease pebrine to microorganisms, and eventually over the validity of germ theory. Béchamp also disputed cell theory.

Claiming discovery that the "molecular granulations" in biological fluids were actually the elementary units of life, Béchamp named them microzymas—that is, "tiny enzymes"—and credited them with producing both enzymes and cells while "evolving" amid favorable conditions into multicellular organisms. Denying that bacteria could invade a healthy animal and cause disease, Béchamp claimed instead that unfavorable host and environmental conditions destabilize the host's native microzymas, whereupon they decompose host tissue by producing pathogenic bacteria. While cell theory and germ theory gained widespread acceptance, granular theories became obscure. Béchamp's version, microzymian theory, has been retained by small groups, especially in alternative medicine.

Why Was There Such A Rivalry Between Pasteur and Bechamp?

In the 19th century France, while Pasteur was advocating the notion of germs as the cause of disease, another French scientist named Antoine Bechamp advocated a conflicting theory known as the "cellular theory" of disease.

Nurturing yourself is not selfish – it's essential to your survival and your well-being."

Renee Peterson Trudeau

Antoine Bechamp (1816-1908) had an incredible list of scientist appointments at French universities: Doctor of Science, Doctor of Medicine, Professor of Medical Chemistry and Pharmacy at Montpelier, Professor of Physics and Toxicology at Strasbourg. The list goes on and on.

During his lifetime Bechamp was overshadowed by the iconic chemist Louis Pasteur (1822-1895), the most celebrated scientist of the nineteenth century. He is considered the Father of Medical Microbiology. And some call him the Father of Modern Medicine, a title quite remarkable as Pasteur was not a physician. Both men were highly-regarded members of the French Academy of Science, and each submitted their scientific findings to the Academy for review and publication.

Because Bechamp frequently criticized Pasteur's work, an intense rivalry and feud between the two intensified in the Academy. But no matter how carefully Bechamp argued against some of Pasteur's scientific methods and conclusions, the Academy always gave the nod to Pasteur.

Bechamp's cellular theory is almost completely opposite to that of Pasteur's. Bechamp noted that these germs that Pasteur was so terrified of were opportunistic in nature. They were everywhere and even existed inside of us in a symbiotic relationship. Bechamp noticed in his research that it was only when the tissue of the host became damaged or compromised that these germs began to manifest as a prevailing symptom (not cause) of disease.

To prevent illness, Bechamp advocated not the killing of germs but the cultivation of health through diet, hygiene, and healthy lifestyle practices such as fresh air and exercise.

82

"What the public expects and what is healthy for an individual are two very different things."

Esther Williams

The idea is that if the person has a strong immune system and good tissue quality (or "terrain" as Bechamp called it), the germs will not manifest in the person, and they will have good health. It is only when their health starts to decline (due to personal neglect and poor lifestyle choices) that they become victim to infections.

You can see this when a group of people goes hiking in the woods. It often seems that the mosquitoes attack only one or two people out of the group. And as it turns out, it's always the same person that always gets attacked by the mosquitoes. This person is usually the one who always catches the latest flu and has the weakest immune system. This is because these germs (including insects) are opportunistic in nature and only attack the weak.

To treat illness, Bechamp's cellular theory also applied. Bechamp was less concerned with killing the infection and focused more on restoring the health of the patient's body through healthy lifestyle choices. Bechamp saw the infection as a footnote to the state of illness and not the primary cause. As the person restored health through diet, hygiene, and detoxification the infection went away on its own—without needing measures to kill it.

Pasteur and Bechamp had a long and often bitter rivalry regarding who was right about the true cause of illness. Ultimately Pasteur's ideas were accepted by society and Bechamp was pretty much forgotten. The practice of Western medicine is based on Pasteur's germ phobia which gives rise to the use of vaccinations, antibiotics, and other anti-microbials.

The irony is that towards the end of his life, Pasteur renounced the germ theory and admitted that Bechamp was right all along. In the 1920's medical historians also discovered that most of Pasteur's theories were plagiarized from Bechamp's early research work.

"Medicine is about disease and what makes people die.

Chiropractic is about life and what makes people live".

B. J. Palmer

What Is The Real Truth Behind The Human Body Around Germs?

Germs are tiny organisms which are so small they cannot be seen without the help of a special instrument called a microscope. The microscope allows the germs to be seen by making them look a lot bigger. Germs are so small and ubiquitous that they creep into our bodies without being noticed.

The human genome is made up of about 23,000 genes. That's a fairly impressive figure until you consider this: the number of non-human genes, each of us carries around, from the bacteria, viruses and other pathogens living in and on us, totals 8 million. Most of the cells in the human body aren't even human. Indeed, bacterial cells outnumber human cells 3 to 1. Which is why the exploration of the human microbiome, the collective population of all the non-human cells and genes that inhabit us, is currently one of the fastest rising fields of medical research.

What scientists are discovering is that these microbes are not just freeloaders or invaders. Rather, they're crucial facilitators of many of our basic bodily functions: from digesting food and producing vitamins to fending off harmful infection and recovering from illness. They not only keep people healthy, but they may also explain differences in individual health — why people respond differently to the same drug or why some people develop chronic diseases and others don't.

Food, water or air can be made dangerous to humans and other animals by things which are living in it or mixed into it. When this happens, it is said to be contaminated or polluted. Food and water can be contaminated by disease-causing germs.

"It is health that is real wealth and not pieces of gold and silver."

Mahatma Gandhi

Germs can get into the body through the mouth, nose, breaks in the skin, eyes, and genitals . Once disease-causing germs are inside the body, they can prevent it from working properly. They may breed very quickly, and in a very short time a small number of germs can become millions.

Lastly, there are many germs inside the human body which may not cause disease. There are even some germs which help parts of the body to work properly. The gut, for example, cannot digest food properly without the help of certain good bacteria.

"When wealth is lost, nothing is lost; when health is lost, something is lost; when character is lost, all is lost."

Billy Graham

CHAPTER 4

The Health Model vs. the Sick Model

One important and positive way that health care is changing is that it's moving from a "sick care" model to a "well care" model. What does this mean? Well, in years past, most health care was provided on a reactive basis. Meaning when you got sick, you went to the doctor; this is the "sick care" model. Today healthcare is moving toward a "well care" model, in which a proactive approach is taken instead, through an ongoing relationship with a primary care practitioner (PCP).

The Health Model (also known as the wellness model) is a theory in caring for clients and patients that takes the focus from being sick to preventative care. In the wellness model, there is a strong emphasis on holistic care where the client or patient is encouraged to take part in healthy activities that create a stronger body and mind that can ward off illness, instead of relying on the traditional health system to care for a sick bodyafter the fact. Wellness is not just a set of practices that are incorporated at the doctor's office, but rather it's a change in lifestyle. Wellness includes care from your regular physician but also can include chiropractic, massage, nutrition, fitness and mental health care. All of these things make you a healthier person.

Health Care vs. Sick Care

Health care is wellness. It's everything that helps you move towards health and prevent problems from occurring again or even in the first place. This includes things like nutrition, exercise, whole food supplements, dental care, chiropractic care, massage, and acupuncture.

"Use your health, even to the point of wearing it out. That is what it is for. Spend all you have before you die; do not outlive yourself."

George Bernard Shaw

Think of it this way. Imagine a spectrum. Health is on one end of the spectrum, and sickness is on the other end of the spectrum. Your position on this spectrum can shift toward one side or the other depending on several factors. On the health end of the spectrum, the focus is on prevention and being proactive in doing things to promote and support health. On the sick end, the focus is on addressing the crisis and being reactive to the disease or illness.

Sick care is damage control. The obvious need for "sick care" is in emergency situations, such as accidents, traumas, and other life-or-death acute conditions. Management of chronic conditions like heart disease, cancer, and diabetes is also included in "sick care." The main goal of "sick care" is to stop you from getting worse. The secondary goal is to make you feel better but not necessarily correct the cause of your problem. The "sick care" model rarely focuses on moving you back towards health and preventing the problem from occurring again.

The Wellness Approach

Wellness care seeks to turn on the natural healing ability, not by adding something to the system, but by removing anything that might interfere with normal function, trusting that the body would know what to do if nothing were interfering with it. Standard medical care, on the other hand, seeks to treat a symptom by adding something from the outside - a medication, a surgery or procedure.

Wellness is a state of optimal conditions for normal function... and then some. The wellness approach is to look for underlying causes of any disturbance or disruption (which may or may not be causing symptoms at the time) and make whatever interventions and lifestyle adjustments would optimize the conditions for normal function.

"There is no effect without a cause. Chiropractors adjust causes. Others treat effects".

B. J. Palmer

That environment encourages natural healing, and minimizes the need for invasive treatment, which should be administered only when absolutely necessary. When the body is working properly, it tends to heal effectively, no matter what the condition. When the body heals well and maintains itself well, then there is another level of health that goes beyond "asymptomatic" or "pain-free" which reveals an open-ended opportunity for vitality, vibrant health, and an enhanced experience of life. This is true for mental and emotional health as well as physical health. While some people may suffer psychological disorders, creating an atmosphere of mental and emotional wellness will address all but the most serious problems.

The Concepts Of Illness Behavior And Sick-Role Behavior In Healthcare

Generally, health-related behaviors of healthy people and those who try to maintain their health are considered as behaviors related to primary prevention of disease. Such behaviors are intended to reduce susceptibility to disease, as well as to reduce the effects of chronic diseases when they occur in the individual. Secondary prevention of disease is more closely related to the control of a disease that an individual has or that is incipient in the individual. This type of prevention is most closely tied to illness behavior. Tertiary prevention is generally seen as directed towards reducing the impact and progression of symptomatic disease in the individual. This type of prevention is highly related to the concept of sick-role behavior.

In present-day public health practice, which is based on population and community-based approaches with an emphasis on participation, the research from these concepts of behavior has helped immensely in clarifying critical approaches to public health. The concept of diversity in populations has been greatly enhanced through the articulation of the concepts of illness behavior and the sick role.

"There's nothing more important than our good health –

that's our principal capital asset."

Arlen Specter

Researchers now have a significant body of research showing the wide variation in these behaviors with respect to all the key demographic variables. For example, there has been excellent work showing how the presentation of symptoms to a physician is highly dependent on gender, ethnic background, and other socio-cultural characteristics. Research on the sick-role concept has elucidated the issue of power and its many manifestations in doctors' offices, hospitals, and other medical settings. It would be difficult, given this literature, for a practicing health educator not to consider the role of power in patient-physician interactions.

In general, illness and sick-role behaviors are viewed as characteristics of individuals and as concepts derived from sociological and socio-psychological theories.

Illness Behavior

The concept of illness behavior was largely defined and adopted during the second half of the twentieth century. Broadly speaking, it is any behavior undertaken by an individual who feels ill to relieve that experience or to better define the meaning of the illness experience. There are many different types of illness behavior that have been studied. Some individuals who experience physical or mental symptoms turn to the medical care system for help; others may turn to self-help strategies; while others may decide to dismiss the symptoms. In everyday life, illness behavior may be a mixture of behavioral decisions. For example, an individual faced with recurring symptoms of joint pain may turn to complementary or alternative medicine for relief. However, sudden, sharp, debilitating symptoms may lead one directly to a hospital emergency room. In any event, illness behavior is usually mediated by strong subjective interpretations of the meaning of symptoms. As with any type of human behavior, many social and psychological factors intervene and determine the type of illness behavior expressed in the individual.

"Health is the greatest of all possessions; a pale cobbler is better than a sick king."

Isaac Bickerstaff

The Health Belief Model

The Health Belief Model (HBM) was developed in the early 1950s by social scientists at the U.S. Public Health Service in order to understand the failure of people to adopt disease prevention strategies or screening tests for the early detection of disease. Later uses of HBM were for patients' responses to symptoms and compliance with medical treatments. The HBM suggests that a person's belief in a personal threat of an illness or disease together with a person's belief in the effectiveness of the recommended health behavior or action will predict the likelihood the person will adopt the behavior.

The Health Belief Model is a framework for motivating people to take positive health actions that uses the desire to avoid a negative health consequence as the prime motivation. For example, HIV is a negative health consequence, and the desire to avoid HIV can be used to motivate sexually active people into practicing safe sex. Similarly, the perceived threat of a heart attack can be used to motivate a person with high blood pressure into exercising more often.

It's important to note that avoiding a negative health consequence is a key element of the HBM. For example, a person might increase exercise to look good and feel better. That example does not fit the model because the person is not motivated by a negative health outcome — even though the health action of getting more exercise is the same as for the person who wants to avoid a heart attack.

The HBM derives from psychological and behavioral theory with the foundation that the two components of health-related behavior are the desire to avoid illness, or conversely get well if already ill; and the belief that a specific health action will prevent, or cure, illness.

"Good health and good sense are two of life's greatest blessings."

Publilius Syrus

Ultimately, an individual's course of action often depends on the person's perceptions of the benefits and barriers related to health behavior. There are six constructs of the HBM.

Perceived Susceptibility: This refers to a person's subjective perception of the risk of acquiring an illness or disease. There is wide variation in a person's feelings of personal vulnerability to an illness or disease.

Perceived Severity: This refers to a person's feelings on the seriousness of contracting an illness or disease (or leaving the illness or disease untreated). There is wide variation in a person's feelings of severity, and often a person considers the medical consequences (e.g., death, disability) and social consequences (e.g., family life, social relationships) when evaluating the severity.

Perceived Benefits: This refers to a person's perception of the effectiveness of various actions available to reduce the threat of illness or disease (or to cure illness or disease). The course of action a person takes in preventing (or curing) illness or disease relies on consideration and evaluation of both perceived susceptibility and perceived benefit, such that the person would accept the recommended health action if it was perceived as beneficial.

Perceived Barriers: This refers to a person's feelings on the obstacles to performing a recommended health action. There is wide variation in a person's feelings of barriers, or impediments, which lead to a cost/benefit analysis. The person weighs the effectiveness of the actions against the perceptions that it may be expensive, dangerous (e.g., side effects), unpleasant (e.g., painful), time-consuming, or inconvenient.

Cue To Action: This is the stimulus needed to trigger the decision-making process to accept a recommended health action.

"INNATE is God in human beings. INNATE is good in human beings. INNATE cannot be cheated, violated, or tricked. INNATE is always waiting, ready to communicate with you, and when INNATE is in contact you are in tune with the Infinite".

B. J. Palmer

These cues can be internal (e.g., chest pains, wheezing, etc.) or external (e.g., advice from others, illness of family member, newspaper article, etc.).

Self-Efficacy: This refers to the level of a person's confidence in his or her ability to successfully perform a behavior. This construct was added to the model most recently in mid-1980's. Self-efficacy is a construct in many behavioral theories as it directly relates to whether a person performs the desired behavior.

Limitations of Health Belief Model

There are several limitations of the HBM which limit its utility in public health. Limitations of the model include the following:

- It does not account for a person's attitudes, beliefs, or other individual determinants that dictate a person's acceptance of a health behavior.

- It does not take into account behaviors that are habitual and thus may inform the decision-making process to accept a recommended action (e.g., smoking).

- It does not take into account behaviors that are performed for non-health related reasons such as social acceptability.

- It does not account for environmental or economic factors that may prohibit or promote the recommended action.

- It assumes that everyone has access to equal amounts of information on the illness or disease.

- It assumes that cues to action are widely prevalent in encouraging people to act and that "health" actions are the main goal in the decision-making process.

"The health of the people is really the foundation upon which all their happiness and all their powers as a state depend."

Benjamin Disraeli

The HBM is more descriptive than explanatory, and does not suggest a strategy for changing health-related actions. In preventive health behaviors, early studies showed that perceived susceptibility, benefits, and barriers were consistently associated with the desired health behavior; perceived severity was less often associated with the desired health behavior. The individual constructs are useful, depending on the health outcome of interest, but for the most effective use of the model, it should be integrated with other models that account for the environmental context and suggest strategies for change.

Preventative Healthcare

Health is a state of wholeness in which your body knows its ever-changing needs and responds to those, all on its own. Inside Out Chiropractic believes that chiropractic care is a long-term form of preventative healthcare that maintains your body's nervous system to keep you in good health for a lifetime.

True chiropractic care in a principled practice believes that bodily health exists when the body is in a state of wholeness; it understands its own constantly-changing needs, and is able to respond to them on its own. Chiropractic care doesn't heal injuries; rather, it helps the body to engage its own incredible natural healing abilities through a long-term routine of preventative healthcare maintenance for the nervous system.

Preventative healthcare focuses on your entire nervous system: your brain, spinal cord, and every one of the millions of nerve connections throughout your body. It monitors your entire body and all its needs, to help control and coordinate the necessary responses that allow the body to learn, adapt and constantly maintain its own health and wellness.

"You can't take good health for granted."

Jack Osbourne

Preventative Care Vs. Sick Care

The common healthcare model in the United States is the sick care model. It only looks at your body after symptoms of illness present, and then considers how best to treat these symptoms.

The preventative healthcare chiropractic model, on the other hand, is entirely natural, non-invasive, doesn't rely on chemicals, and looks to the root cause of your underlying health issues. It is focused entirely on correcting spinal subluxations to allow your whole nervous system to communicate better and increase the body's overall healing abilities. This improves your ability to adapt to stress and a variety of health conditions and helps to restore you to normal, healthy and optimal function. Chiropractic can restore your natural healing capability, and provide increased vitality, energy, bodily functions and overall health.

Hospitals and the Wellness Sham

Furthermore, while hospitals and health systems may preach wellness, few offer comprehensive services designed to improve your health and well-being. Rather, they pay lip-service to this essential component of health care – viewing wellness more as a marketing opportunity than a true effort to do everything in their power to minimize unnecessary and costly utilization of their medical services.

There's no surprise here, since the dominant reimbursement mechanism, the fee for service, rewards the provision of medical services – not maximization of the health of a defined population. As a result, we pay a very dear price.

"Get Health. No labor, effort nor exercise that can gain it
must be grudged."

Ralph Waldo Emerson

How to Move from Sickness to Wellness

This can be a big challenge for some of our clients. And the reality is, moving from a sickness state of mind to a wellness state of mind is incredibly personal. It is possible to shift from a sick-care system that doles out interventions to manage the burden of chronic illness to a positive health system, focused on wellness/well-being system that minimizes unnecessary utilization by focusing on population health. However, it would reQuire tremendous will on the part of numerous constituents to achieve such a powerful transformation.

The key to transitioning from one model to the other is time and support. When we meet a new client who can benefit from the wellness model, we address their immediate issues, and then create a positive and encouraging atmosphere that they can feel comfortable expanding into. If they've come to see us for chiropractic care, we may encourage them to support that function with a visit to one of our massage therapists or a fitness class. Treating the whole body with kindness and mindfulness is often all it takes to move a client from being "sick" to being "well."

Far short of transformational change, there are nonetheless small seeds of hope in the form of new, evolving reimbursement and delivery models, such as ACOs and medical homes that stress population health management. Unfortunately, the pace of adoption is glacial. For providers who have been burned in the past by assuming the risk for a defined population, there's little enthusiasm for doing so again.

Our Role in Changing the System

More than three decades ago, Jim Fries gave us one of the keys to healing American health care; a silver bullet.

"Nature needs no help, just no interference".

B. J. Palmer

The question is whether we have the fortitude to change the healthcare paradigm, as well as accept the personal, stewardship responsibility for our health that is essential to success. Below are the roles for each of us to play:

Government: There needs to be dramatically increased spending on proven prevention programs that can be administered at a local, state, or federal level. Furthermore, there need to be greater rewards under governmental reimbursement programs for those providers who embrace risk and demonstrate their ability to reduce the morbidity of a defined population.

Consumers/Patients: We need to understand what it means to be prudent stewards of our health, and the health of our families. It is essential that we understand the role lifestyle choices make in determining our health, and how we might combat risk-factors that imperil our future. For many of us, we will need to have access to resources that will aid in this journey – particularly if we are socio-economically challenged, and thus find lifestyle change all the more difficult. As has been well-demonstrated, the social determinants of health play a profound role in wellness and well-being.

Providers: Healthcare executives need to take the moral high-ground and do the right things for the communities they serve. One place to begin is with the development of a strategic wellness plan illustrating how wellness initiatives can be integrated into the very fabric of your hospital or health system's care model. Once developed and implemented, you can then reasonably assert that you do everything possible to minimize unnecessary consumption of health care resources while maximizing the health and well-being of your patients.

"Your body hears everything your mind says."

Naomi Judd

Insurers/Payers: There needs to be an unremitting pressure to partner more fully with providers on the assumption of risk for the health and well-being of a defined population, thus accelerating the demise of fee-for-service medicine, and its replacement with a reimbursement mechanism that rewards wellness.

Employers: There needs to be broader adoption and implementation of wellness programs that incorporate proven mechanisms for elevating the health and well-being of an employed population. Such programs will likely involve potent incentives for lifestyle modification by those employees at risk.

Conclusion

It's time to put the "health" back in healthcare. Physicians must join with other health care practitioners whose focus is on building health and wellness and not just managing disease and illness. Drugs and surgeries target the main complaint and symptoms. But they fail to address the cause of the problems plaguing current day society. No amount of medication will address the true cause of degenerative diseases if the dysfunction within the body is not identified and restored. The irony is that the majority of the top 10 causes of death in modern society are rooted in diet and lifestyle (heart disease, certain cancers, diabetes, Alzheimer's – to name a few). These conditions may never have grown to their current epic proportions if the medical community would have continued to honor the fundamental health building values of diet and exercise.

"Take care of your body with steadfast fidelity. The soul must see through these eyes alone, and if they are dim, the whole world is clouded."

Johann Wolfgang von Goethe

CHAPTER 5

APPRECIATING THE MARVEL OF HUMAN LIFE

Before I begin to discuss anything else, I want to take this chapter to begin to appreciate this thing called human life. Appreciating the astounding way in which our human body works. I am not talking about something mystical, instead asking you to think about the complexities of our body, and isn't it marvelous that we exist in the first place.

Just think about our body that is made of billions and billions of cells working in sync with each other, the heart that beats untiringly 100, 000 times a day, our breath, and senses send millions of signals each day. Blood vessels extending to thousands of miles, and yet at the end of the day not a single breakdown. So the key to changing our life is by first appreciating it.

Our life is marvelous, considering that the chances of us being alive are just 1 in 75 million!

I know it's hard to believe, but it's true. Only 1 in 75 million sperms get a chance to fertilize the egg. But things are not that simple, considering that females ovulate just once a month, and the ovum survives on average just 72 hours. Furthermore, many of the fertilized eggs just fail to establish themselves in the uterus before the start of a woman's period, thus resulting in failure of pregnancy. So how is it possible that with all of these complexities that we still exist? The answer is simple; our DNA has much more information and power than most in the scientific world can even imagine.

"Your body holds deep wisdom. Trust in it. Learn from it. Nourish it. Watch your life transform and be healthy."

Bella Bleue

DNA contains all the information, and instructions, controlling the growth, maturity, and daily functioning of each and every cell in our body. It controls how the cells should behave together making a particular kind of tissue or organ be it heart, liver, skin, or muscles.

Since the decoding of DNA, we know a lot about how it works. How this small bundle can control most things, and how the smallest error in its functioning can lead to diseases. Scientists are just starting to unravel and appreciate the power of DNA.

Only a small active part of our DNA makes us what we are, and most of the DNA is dormant. It is the role of this dormant part that researchers are trying to unravel.

DNA is coded quite like a spoken language, with its own set of rules, similar to the grammar rules of language we speak. Meaning, DNA has a role to play in a way we speak, and on the other hand, words and thoughts have the power to influence the DNA itself, something long mentioned in spiritual science, but now being discovered by the modern science.

It means that DNA can be modified by using vibrations and suggestions, thus explaining how the power of intention and beliefs can heal our body, and have a potent effect on our mind.

In fact, researchers in Russia are redefining the role of DNA in quantum science, space, and relative theories. Researchers think that DNA has the power to propagate information independent of space and time. Meaning that with the help of DNA we can communicate, and create a huge communication group, researchers are exploring such possibilities in a Global Consciousness Project. Though it is too early to say about the effect of such hyper communicating group on our existence, but DNA would surely have a central role in it.

"Have you more faith in a spoonful of medicine than in the power that animates the living world?"

B. J. Palmer

"The information stored in DNA must by no means be underestimated. So much so that one human DNA molecule contains enough information to fill a million-page encyclopedia, or to fill about 1,000 books."

-HARUN YABYA author of ETERNITY HAS ALREADY BEGUN

Thus the first step to good health is to appreciate the power of DNA, appreciate how the fusion of just two cells transformed into 70 trillion cells by the time of birth.

Everything is marvelous about the way we take shape from the day one. Our brain is the first organ that starts forming; then it is covered by the bony shield we call a skull in adults, after which our spinal cord, the powerful information highway starts developing. Only once the central computing and information highway is ready that other body parts and organs start taking shape. The autonomic nervous system takes over the control of our internal organs, ensuring that heart beats as intended, digestive juices are secreted as required.

I am not trying to teach you human anatomy, but just to underline the intricacies of the human body. Emphasizing the importance of the nervous system, and how it controls the functioning of each and every cell, playing a crucial role in health maintenance by responding to every challenge.

However, if our nervous system somehow fails to respond to these daily challenges suitably, balance is broken. Yes, you got it, it leads to disease. So you must be asking that in what way can I take control this process.

So summarizing all this in one sentence, just remember that: *Doctor's don't cure, the body cures itself.*

"There is no one giant step that does it. It's a lot of little steps."

Unknown

Thus the good doctor is one who adopts a holistic approach, appreciates the flow of the healing power inside each of us. However, there aren't many such doctors, simply because medical schools don't teach all this. Thus it's all up to you!

So what I want you to do right now is to thank your body in serving you in such a beautiful manner, appreciate your body for your existing, respect it for doing all the wonderful things for your existence. Respect and appreciate the abilities of your body, and treat it as most wonderful thing you have ever owned.

Its time that you realize what a wonderful gift your body is, there is a reason for you being here. You cannot get a kind of life you want without a true connection to the importance of your wellbeing. Start today with a new gratitude that your life requires true energy, not just a halfhearted effort, rather aim for the maximum you have ever desired.

INNATE INTELLIGENCE AND THE BODY'S FUNCTIONS

As I already mentioned earlier that it all started with a single cell, but how that single cell transformed into the massive body? Miracle?

Well, not exactly, it is what Chiropractors are calling *Innate Intelligence* for more than a century. It is something that is created at the moment of your inception; it flows through your body, it is what makes your body function in a way it should be functioning without a glitch. Our body is a wonder of Innate Intelligence. It operates automatically. It does everything from maintaining your heart rhythm to keeping your skin supple.

"I have chosen to be happy because it is good for my health."

Voltaire

THE HEART

The heart is one of the sturdiest pumps, though weighing merely 11 ounces, it is just the size of the fist, it is made up of the strongest muscles in our body, and at the same time, it has tissues that are more delicate than tissue paper. These delicate tissues have neurons that make up almost half of the heart. Yes, the same tissues that make up the nervous system and spine.

The beating of the heart creates powerful electromagnetic impulses; it is these impulses that are registered by an apparatus called the ECG. They flow to and from the heart in a torus. The torus is a shape similar to a donut. This torus stretches from the top of the head till the pelvic floor.

The torus-shaped field is present not only in the heart, in fact, all molecules have a torus-like electromagnetic field. Thus we are able to connect with the rest of our body and the world around us. If a person is ill, it makes the heart susceptible.

Each cell of our heart communicates with each other and work in synchrony with each other. This synchronous action of heart muscles helps to supply 6000 quarts of blood each day covering the distance of 60 000 miles through arteries and veins.

The heart never stops or takes breaks, it is simple, yet one of the most critical parts of our body that functions to bring oxygen from the lungs and deliver it to the rest of the body.

THE LUNGS

Lungs are another brilliant example of innate intelligence at work. The primary function of lungs is to keep your body oxygenated, remove carbon dioxide and other wastes of metabolism.

"Health is a state of body. Wellness is a state of being."

J. Stanford

During inhalation, our rib cage expands to allow maximum air inside, while during exhalation rib cage becomes smaller to push out the air. Ribs are quite dynamic, and muscles between them are flexible, allowing air to flow in and out of the lungs.

When air enters the lungs, it reaches the small sac-like structure called alveoli, where it meets the pulmonary capillaries, and gaseous exchange takes place. Oxygen enters our body, and carbon dioxide is expelled out.

Though automatic, respiration is a highly regulated process, enabling our heart to breath 20-30 000 times a day, working continually under the supervision of the autonomous nervous system.

THE SKIN

Skin is not there just to provide the cover, in fact, it is the largest organ of our body amounting to about 16 percent of total body weight. Apart from protection, it helps to maintain body temperature, remove excess of water, salt, and toxins.

Skin is the first line of defense for our internal organs from every imaginable danger, be it infection or ultraviolet rays. It even converts sun rays to vitamin D and thus helping to maintain healthy bones.

Skin also plays a vital role in communication, sensation, expression of emotions, and even sexual attraction. It is made up of two layers called epidermis and dermis. Skin can also absorb oily substances.

THE DIGESTIVE SYSTEM

It starts from the mouth, from their onwards food reaches the stomach while passing through the pipe called the esophagus. Movement of food in the digestive system happens due to a rhythmic movement called peristalsis, an action that is similar to squeezing from one end till other. It is a brilliant example of innate intelligence at work.

"It takes 65 muscles to frown and 13 to make a smile.

Why work overtime?"

B. J. Palmer

Once food enters our stomach, it is mixed with digestive juices and then passed on to the small intestine, where it is further broken down and processed with pancreatic juices and gallbladder juices.

Digestive system provides the body with all the necessary elements. Carbohydrates are the source of energy, proteins are the building blocks, while fats serve as energy reserves, and are also essential for proper brain function. Minerals and vitamins are needed for complex biochemical processes. The fiber in the diet helps in the movement of food.

When our digestive system is functioning as it should be, we are full of energy, able to fight infections. If we eat a diet poor in ideal nutrients, our health will suffer. If we overeat something, it may also have a negative impact. The body tries to store the excess of calories in the form of fat below the skin.

THE LIVER

The chemical factory of our body is the largest organ inside our body. It produces bile that helps to digest carbs, proteins, and fats. It also helps in building certain proteins.

The liver is also called the garbage can, as it removes toxins from the blood at the same time absorbing fat-soluble vitamins. Liver and kidney are the two organs that remove most of the toxins.

The liver also controls blood sugar levels by storing or releasing them as need be. It works as the blood filter. It is divided into four parts, receiving blood from some of the largest arteries and veins.

THE KIDNEYS

Another vital organ located in the abdominal cavity. We have two of them, and they function as the filters.

"Exercise to have fun and be healthy, not just to lose weight."

Unknown

They help to maintain water and electrolyte balance, regulate pH of the blood, removes toxins from the blood.

Kidneys also play an important role in maintaining the level of vital nutrients in the blood. It also makes vitamin D, produces hormones responsible for regulation of blood pressure, produces a hormone called erythropoietin that stimulates the growth of red blood cells.

We do not care much about kidneys until they develop stones or get hurt by diabetes. Kidney stones are deposition of high levels of calcium, uric acid, and oxalate in urine.

Kidneys play a vital role in regulating osmotic pressure of extracellular fluids, regulation of pH, in maintaining blood pressure, secreting metabolic wastes.

THE EYES

Despite its small size, it is the most important sensory organ, having millions of cells that provide the sense of sight. Although eyes can perceive only red, yellow, blue, and black, it can differentiate between 300 trillion colors!

Sitting in the bony socket of the skull, it has a lens to focus light on the sensor called the retina. The retina sends visual information to the brain with the help of optical nerves. The small colored portion in the center of the eyes called the iris, controls the amount of light that can enter inside the eye. In bright light the pupil contracts, while in low light conditions they dilate to allow more light into the eyes.

Eyes are protected by eyelids and eyelashes. They blink on a regular interval to keep the upper layer of eyes moist.

All these activities in the eyes happen automatically due to innate intelligence.

"Health is a state of complete physical, mental and social well-being and not merely the absence of disease or infirmity."

World Health Organization

THE HAND

We are the only species with opposing fingers and thumbs, this amazing instrument is powered by 13 muscles, and has 27 bones for extra flexibility. It can carry out very delicate jobs like playing the keyboard to participating in rigorous sports.

The wrist, though not a part of the hand is made up of eight carpals, and anyone suffering from carpal tunnel knows about them.

A chiropractor is especially good at understanding and treating the pain related to carpal tunnel syndrome. As an example, one of my clients who already had an operation for this condition came to me, as the pain was not relieved by surgery. I could see that the pain of the client was due to a problem in the neck.

After carpals, comes the metacarpals, forming the palm, then comes the phalanges, 14 small bones forming the fingers and thumbs. The thumbs have just two phalanges, while each finger has three of them.

Metacarpals are joints to the phalanges with joints called MIPs, while joints in fingers are called PIP (proximal interphalangeal joint), and DIP (distal interphalangeal joint).

If you are confused with the structure of the hand, don't worry, that is just to demonstrate the complexity of the subject. What is important is that you appreciate how innate intelligence controls this complex structure.

THE EARS

It is this amazing organ that makes enjoying music possible, due to them we can hear the sweet laughter of our children. The ear is divided into the outer, middle, and inner ear.

"Health is the thing that makes you feel that now is the best time of year."
Franklin P. Adams

Two important components that make hearing possible are air conduction and bone conduction.

Airwaves move through the ear canal and hit the eardrum. Another name for the ear drum is the"tympanic membrane," this membrane vibrates like a huge drum after being hit.

The vibration of the eardrum causes the movement of the small bones inside the ear. These bones called the malleus, incus, and stapes are the smallest bones in the body. As the stapes vibrates, it causes the movement of the fluid in the inner ear.

The inner year also contains the cochlea where the hearing takes place. The cochlea contains thousands of hairy structures that move along with the fluid of internal ear, thus generating the electrical signal sent to the brain through auditory nerve.

Another way of hearing is bone conduction, when loud vibrations are conducted through the skull, it makes our inner ear fluid vibrate.

THE MUSCLES

There are whopping 650 of them in our body, making all of our movements possible. They are made to do most complicated tasks like picking small objects with tweezers to more robust tasks like running a marathon. Muscles also help to protect the internal organs.

Though we may know a lot about the functioning of our muscles, but in reality, things are more complicated. To perform any tasks, muscles must work in synchronization with various other organs. Thus moving from one place to another involves communication between muscles, ears, eyes, and brain. All this happens by using the information highway called our nervous system.

"Every organ in your body is connected to the one under your hat".

B. J. Palmer

When our muscles and joints are moving, all the information about actions, movement, location is being transmitted to the brain at a subconscious level, a communication being controlled by innate intelligence.

In fact, we do far more tasks than we ever realize. Thus if a person starts talking to you, you automatically turn your head, eyes, and start listening to this person.

It is innate intelligence that makes balancing possible, by controlling the minor muscular movements at all times. Our balance and movement will become sluggish if even one small muscle fails to perform as required. Thus the brain has to keep correcting the movement at all times.

It must be understood that motion or movement caused by contraction of muscles does not include just movement of the body from one point to another, but it also includes heartbeats, breathing, movements in glands, movements of all the visceral organs, movement of blood and lymph. Thus muscular contraction is responsible for controlling various physiological activities.

THE SKELETAL SYSTEM

Without bones we would be just an enormous blob with no shape or structure, we would not be able to stand or walk. Without bones, we would be just a pile of skin, muscles, and guts.

Our skeletal system is made up of 206 bones, designed to be strong, and to protect our body. At birth we have 300 bones, but as we grow many of them fuse together.

Bones have many functions. The spinal vertebrae not only protects the information highway but also helps us to stand erect and walk upright. Bones protect the delicate internal organs.

"Embrace and love your body. It's the most amazing thing you will ever own."

Unknown

Just consider the skull, it's like a strong helmet safeguarding our brain. The rib cage protects our heart and lungs.

Unlike the common perception that bones are cold and inert, they are in fact, very dynamic. Bones are made of a hard layer for providing strength and cells that help them grow and repair. That is why if you have ever broken your arm or leg, it heals.

There are several types of bones. 1). Long bones: they have a central shaft and two extremities. The shaft is made mainly of robust and compact tissue. Long bones have unique curves for providing them with extra strength. 2). Short bones: they are mostly irregular in shape. They are spongy, with only a thin layer of compact tissues. Carpal bones are an example of them. 3). Flat bones: they are not very strong, usually required for the attachment of the muscles. 4). Irregular bones: called so because of their peculiar shape. Bones of the vertebra or those inside the ear are good examples of them.

Apart from mechanical support and protection, bones are also responsible for producing red and white blood cells. Red blood cells are responsible for carrying oxygen to body tissues, while white blood cells are the part of the immune system, thus helping to protect our body from infections and diseases.

ONCE AGAIN... THE NERVOUS SYSTEM

We once again return to discuss the system that controls our majestic body- the nervous system. It consists of the brain, spinal cord, and peripheral nerves. The brain is the main computing center that sends signals to various parts of the body, performing billions of operations and yet consuming merely around ten watts of energy. The spinal cord is the information "Superhighway," that is responsible for distributing all the information. Spinal nerves are the exit points of the highway.

"Wellness Encompasses a healthy body, a sound mind, and a tranquil spirit. Enjoy the journey as you strive for wellness."

Laurette Gagnon Beaulieu

The nervous system is operated by innate intelligence that is vital for the functioning of every cell. And most of the time it efficiently performs its tasks to ensure that the body works in tandem. Innate intelligence can be called the "internal divine guidance," that overlooks all the critical function to ensure the proper health.

Any disruption in communication between the body parts and the brain would lead to either pain or a loss of functionality. It is like a disruption in the telephone line which makes communication between the two parties compromised.

Thus for optimal health, it is vital that our nervous system is working correctly all the time to maintain hundred percent communication throughout the body. In this chapter, we demonstrated that our body is made up of various systems that operate in synchronization with each other to ensure optimal health.

THE MIRACLE OF LIFE

Each day thousands of babies come into this world, take their first breath, and yet nothing can explain what is making this miracle a reality. In medical terms a fetus is called a baby after 20 weeks of pregnancy. By 20 weeks, most of its organs are fully formed, it starts making movements, can even suck its thumb, and all that is visible on ultrasound. It is attached to the wall of the womb by the placenta and umbilical cord. The umbilical cord is connected to the baby's belly button, two arteries and a vein pass through this umbilical cord, feeding the baby and carrying away the waste products.

The baby can urinate but does not have bowel movements until birth. Surrounding amniotic fluid in the womb is circulated every five hours to ensure a safe and clean environment for the baby.

"The only way to keep your health is to eat what you don't want, drink what you don't like, and do what you'd rather not."

Mark Twain

The temperature is maintained continuously at 98.6 F. The amniotic fluid also works as a shock absorber to prevent trauma to the tender organism.

The primary function of the placenta is a metabolic and gaseous exchange between the mother and the baby; it also produces hormones. In the early stages of development, the placenta is made up of four layers, but by the fourth month only two layers are left, thus ensuring the fastest exchange of nutrients. Well, that is enough detail to give you an idea of how miraculous the environment inside the womb is.

Then comes the miraculous day, a day to descend into the outside world. The amniotic membrane breaks and the baby slowly squeezes out of the mother. The doctor would help the baby in coming out. Once out, the baby may sometimes need stimulus. And then comes the first cry. No one can tell what makes the baby take that first breath; it is a miracle, a mystery that is repeated thousands of time each day around the world.

From the very first breath, you are a marvel! Now that you are aware that YOU are a marvel, it is your duty to take care of your health. It is comical that most people do not see themselves as a marvel, thus they don't care about their wellbeing, and unfortunately, they continue to harm their body.

"Knowledge is knowing a fact, wisdom is knowing what to do with that fact".

B. J. Palmer

Chapter 6

The History of Chiropractic

The history of healthcare in the United states is much brighter and diverse than most think. In the latter part of the 19th Century, Medical care was dominated by two schools of thought: The School of Homeopathy and the School of Eclecticism, which had supplanted the traditional medical practices of the day which consisted of mainly bloodletting, sometimes by means of leaches, and metallic poisoning by means of mercury and arsenic in what were considered to be therapeutic doses. In 1847 , the American Medical Association was established to attempt to regulate the industry as until that time there were no licensing requirements or standard practices, nor even standardized educational requirements. Up until that time anyone could could open up shop as a doctor and the open market was left to determine their success or failure. By the beginning of the 20th century, most states had adopted medical licensing laws and standard curriculum requirements.

It was at this time, while the traditional therapies tended to be very dangerous, that Magnetic healing began to be popular as an alternative form of health care, not involving metal poisoning or bloodletting. Magnetic healing does not, as the name implies, involve the use of magnets, but rather the "magnetism" and personality of the practitioner who would heal the patient through the use of subtle suggestion and oftentimes hypnotherapy. One of these magnetic healers, a man named D.D. Palmer, had discovered, quite by accident, that manipulation of the spine, or rather corrective repositioning of the vertebrae could have a positive effect on the health of the patient.

"To insure good health: eat lightly, breathe deeply, live moderately, cultivate cheerfulness, and maintain an interest in life."

William Londen

This idea wasn't new. In 1892, Dr Andrew Taylor Still had formed the American School of Osteopathy in Kirksville, MO. This discipline stressed the importance of proper bone alignment to the flow of vital fluids, or "humors" of the body. The concept was that interruption of proper flow resulted in stagnation of the body and the conditions of illness.

The difference was that D.D. Palmer became convinced that the it was the proper flow of information through the nervous system that ensured health, and that bio mechanical interference's in "nerve flow"caused disease states or what he referred to as "dis-ease". He called the impingments "subluxations" and attributed most health concerns to this condition. In 1895 he had re-positioned a bone in his janitor's back that seemed out of place. The janitor, a certain Harvey Lillard, the much celebrated first Chiropractic patient, reported that it was this bone "popping-out" which had lead to his hearing loss and subsequently upon it's return, the restoration of his hearing. In 1897, Daniel David Palmer founded the first Chiropractic School in Davenport Iowa. In 1906, His son B.J. Palmer took over the school and really began to develop the practice and philosophy of Chiropractic.

At the same time as health care was developing in the United States along these divergent paths, germ theory came into existence. With the advancements in science following the Civil War, most human disease was now beginning to be attributed to germs. Science was finally stepping into the arena and replacing metaphysics as the basis of medical thought and healthcare. The days of morphine, cocaine, and mercury Cure All's were coming to an end. The era of the snake oil salesman was soon to diminish. It hasn't ever yet completely disappeared however.

At this time Dr Still had begun to refer to Chiropractic as a "bastardization of Osteopathy" and in fact D.D. Palmer does make reference in his personal notes to having taken classes in Osteopathy.

"A man too busy to take care of his health is like a

mechanic too busy to take care of his tools."

Spanish Proverb

The medical establishment took a strong opposing view to Chiropractic and regularly sought to punish Chiropractors as falsely practicing medicine. The public was mixed. Early perceptions of Chiropractic were tainted by the Medical establishments disdain for Chiropractors, led by Dr Morris Fishbein the "Medical Mussolini". He began an official AMA effort to discredit Chiropractic, and led it for over fifty years in an attempt to destroy the profession. The AMA founded the "Commission on Quackery" in 1962 and adopted measures to ban medical doctor from having professional affiliations with Chiropractors, and pursue political goals with the intent to discredit and destroy Chiropractic practice. This effort ended in 1987 with the decision on the Wilk's case wherein the AMA was put under permanent injunction to halt anti-Chiropractic activities and forced to print formal apologies and retractions in the Journal of the American Medical Association.

Chiropractic is poised now to take a leading role in the healthcare industry as formal studies are ever increasingly showing it's efficacy in the treatment of musculoskeletal and other disorders, and as a growing faction of the public trends away from pharmaceuticals as appropriate treatment for many conditions and disorders.

Chiropractic is now generally considered to be effective in the treatment of many disorders by a growing sector of the public, and in fact, JMPT published in 2015 a study that shows that a majority of Americans believe Chiropractic is safe an effective for neck or back pain and that Chiropractors were trustworthy as healthcare providers.

Many people now use Chiropractors as the first line or "portal of entry" caregivers when faced with low back or neck pain, headaches, many types of numbness and radiating pain disorders as well as when facing a personal injury or work related injury. Government studies conducted by the Department of Defense have shown that Chiropractic is safe and effective for low back pain and neck pain.

"To keep the body in good health is a duty, for otherwise we shall not be able to trim the lamp of wisdom, and keep our mind strong and clear. Water surrounds the lotus flower, but does not wet its petals."

Buddha

As a matter of fact, this author was one of the first military personnel to be treated in experimental trials in the US Army in 1997, and this was my introduction to Chiropractic. My treatments were for migraine headaches and the results were so impressive as to cause me to change career paths and become a Chiropractor myself.

As my familiarity with Chiropractic grew during the study period, I realized that many other issues were also amenable to Chiropractic care. I had long suffered low back pain and this began to resolve during my treatments, as well as many other aches and pains which I had accumulated through fifteen years of Military service, and thirteen years playing Rugby.

The public, and even the Medical institutions, now generally regard Chiropractic to safe and effective in the treatment of mainly musculoskeletal problems such as low back and neck pain. Many people with experience with Chiropractic care will also attest that it is effective on a myriad of other health issues, some not considered musculoskeletal or bio-mechanical. The concentration of the research however, tends to focus on low back and neck pain and some related neuropathies, so the majority of findings also tend to be in that arena.

Studies funded by the National Institutes for Health showed that 53% of patients realized at least 75% reduction in neck pain while only 33% of patients using pharmaceutical realized that level of relief. Post study at one year, 53% of Chiropractic patients still had at least 75% reduction of pain while the group receiving traditional medical care (pharmaceutical) reported 38% experienced a 75% or greater reduction of pain. Chiropractic is useful in the reduction of many types of neck pain which are due to trauma. A whiplash type injury is essentially a sprained neck, and in order to heal properly the structure must be returned to it's appropriate positioning.

"All the drugs in the world cannot adjust subluxated vertebrae."

B. J. Palmer

When someone suffers a whiplash, which is a very common type of injury in today's world, usually the structures around C%, the middle vertebra in your neck get strained, stretched and torn. The vertebra moves to a posterior position, and the ligaments and tendons cannot heal properly because they are stretched and torn. The only way to let them heal properly is to bring the vertebra back into the proper position so that the ligaments and tendons connected to it can be in the proper place. When this vertebra is out of place, it also distorts the natural curve of the neck, causing the head to be held too far forward. This malposition of the head causes the muscles of the upper back and neck to work overtime trying to support the weight of the head which they are not designed to do. This can cause cramping, shoulder pain and headaches. This malposition can also cause nerves to be stretched and pinched resulting in numbness in the hands and fingers as well as weakness. Many people are improperly diagnosed with carpal tunnel syndrome due to problems that actually lie in their neck. But this is only one example of a neck problem which can be treated by chiropractic. There are many others as a result of the fact that the brain and body connect and communicate through so many complicated structures which lie in the cervical area, or neck. This area is one of the most important areas Chiropractors treat and in fact there are some specialized Chiropractors, generally referred to as "Upper Cervical Chiropractors" who only concentrate on this area and the exhaustive and detailed study of cervical biomechanics and neurology.

Low back pain is another area where chiropractors are known to perform well. Recently the AMA (American Medical Association), the same one who spent untold effort to derail Chiropractic in the early 20th century, has advised officially that patients should always exhaust Chiropractic as an alternative before considering back surgery for low back pain.

"Now there are more overweight people in America than average-weight people. So overweight people are now average. Which means you've met your New Year's resolution."

Jay Leno

About 7.7 million Americans go to Chiropractors for low back pain every year. Treatment for low back pain may consist of spinal manipulations called "adjustments" as well as exercise and stretching programs, biomechanical retraining such as gait (walking) and deep tissue work, electro-therapies and other modalities similar to and including physical therapy. Most low back pain is cause by derangement of the alignment of the lumbar (low back) spine and the subsequent effect it has on the surrounding tissues. Swelling of the surrounding tissues, pinching of nerves and damage to or undo pressure on disks all attribute to low back pain. The causes of low back pain are myriad and complex, as the structure of the low back is complex, and generally supports the weight of the entire body, even allowing movement. There are many different conditions that contribute to or cause low back pain, and even more that can affect radiating pain such as sciatica or Iliotibial syndrome that shoot down the legs. Entire textbooks have been written on this subject and it is beyond the scope of this book to go into them too far. Be assured that your Chiropractor has the education and training to competently address these issues. Chiropractors are specialists and generally know more about the causes and treatments of low back pain than any other profession. Studies show that Chiropractic care for low back pain leads to better recovery, less pain, less relapse, and less risk than other approaches.

As I had previously mentioned, my introduction to Chiropractic care was through the initial studies conducted at Evans Army Hospital at Ft Carson CO when I was put into a study group of patients for the treatment of migraine headaches. This turned out to be a life altering event for me. I had been through uncountable treatment regimens for my headaches in the traditional medical system, and never had any noticeable improvement whatsoever. When I first reported to the Chiropractor, I was skeptical, to say the least. I called him a "Witch Doctor" and let him know that the only reason I was there was because I had no choice. This man's patience with me was immeasurable.

"Don't eat anything your great-great grandmother wouldn't recognize as food. There are a great many food-like items in the supermarket your ancestors wouldn't recognize as food.. stay away from these"

Michael Pollan

He first explained what he was going to do and why. I thought to myself, "well, that's new!" as no medical doctor had ever bothered to try to explain the mechanism of migraine headaches to me before. So I eased up a little and let him do his thing. He adjusted my neck and my persistent headache went away almost immediately. I couldn't believe it. He continued to explain the mechanism that was affecting me specifically, and it made perfect sense. I had always wondered how, whenever I went to a medical doctor concerning my headaches, and I would go through sleep tests, and MRI studies, and PET scans, and blood tests and at the end of the visit when I asked what they had found, they didn't know. They would say that they have to wait for the test results to come back, yet somehow they had a prescription for me! "How can you treat me if you don't know what's wrong?" I wondered. I have since figured it out. The Medical profession was concentrating on treating my headaches, after all that was my complaint. Pain. Pain goes away – no more problem. But the pain didn't go away. This Chiropractor guy – he took a different approach, he figured out what was causing the pain and fixed that instead, and then the pain went away because my body didn't need it anymore. That's right, my body made me perceive pain because it was trying to tell me something, It was a warning light. The medical doctors were concentrating on shutting off the warning light. The Chiropractor was figuring out what the warning light was telling me. That's the difference. That made all the difference. That made Chiropractic look like something completely different to me. It looked honest. It went to the root of the problem. In the army we would refer to doing shoddy work as "paint over rust". That's how we dealt with problems that we didn't really care to solve. Paint over rust, it's good enough for now. By the time it rusts through, it'll be someone else's problem. That's what the medical approach to me and my problem had always been The doctors were painting over my rust and sending me on down the line. When my warning light went on, the answer was to put some electric tape over the light so you couldn't see it.

"Health is a relationship between you and your body"

Terri Guillemets

The Chiropractor inspected the wiring harness and found the short. He fixed the problem. That's why I became a Chiropractor. I won't tell you that all headaches are the same as mine because they're not. I will tell you that most headaches will respond to Chiropractic care. I will also tell you that no headaches are due to pharmaceutical deficiencies, with the exception of withdrawal headaches. As a matter of fact, almost no health conditions at all are due to pharmaceutical deficiencies, except withdrawal and type I diabetes. There are numerous studies that validate chiropractic efficacy for headache treatment, a simple online search will prove that to you.

There are also many other conditions that respond well to chiropractic treatments. Some of them would be carpal tunnel syndrome which is often misdiagnosed. The current surgical procedure of cutting the flexor retinaculum in half has about a 20% long term success rate. The problem that constitutes carpal tunnel syndrome is an anterior dislocation of a bone in your wrist called the Lunate bone. The symptoms arise from that bone pressing on the median nerve in your wrist, in a place called the carpal tunnel, making your fingers go numb. The logical solution: put the lunate bone back in place. The medical solution: cut out the ligament that holds the wrist together and let everything spill out into a position where there is no more pressure. One problem with that approach is that any condition which puts strain on the medial nerve will have the same symptoms. You could have cubital tunnel syndrome, which is in the elbow, you could have tunnel of Guyon syndrome, which is in the wrist but in a different part, or you could have cervical neuropathy where the problem is a strain on the roots of the median nerve in your neck. It could even be a presentation of Thoracic Outlet Syndrome which can be caused by a number of problems in the chest and shoulder area. Once the surgery is done however, it can't be undone.

"Healing is a process afforded you by your Creator and is above and beyond the control of man. Your Chiropractor does everything possible to help Innate heal-but he cannot heal nor can anyone else produce healing for you. When the right adjustment is made, Innate goes to work. You feel the results when dis-ease turns to ease".

B. J. Palmer

Another common problem which responds well to Chiropractic care, but is usually medically treated with surgery that can't be undone is Plantar Fasciitis. This is usually addressed by cutting the plantar fascia, a ligament which is important to the structure of the foot. It is usually a simple matter of repositioning the heel bone, or calcaneous, when it is deviated from it's proper alignment that solves this problem, by correcting the issue which caused it. The patient may also need to begin doing calf stretches or lose weight, or have a gait deficiency which is affecting the foot and causing the bone misalignment, but the problem isn't that the plantar fascia has suddenly shrunk and become too tight and needs to be cut or removed. It's not excess. None of your essential body parts are excess. All of the regular anatomy that you have is supposed to be there. I treat a lot of issues that people don't think a Chiropractor would address. I see a lot of patients who have problems that the regular health care system has misdiagnosed or mistreated or doesn't have an answer for. Many times it is a misunderstanding on the part of conventional medicine that pain is not a condition, it is the way your body tells you that you have a condition. If you only treat the pain, that's like shutting the dog up for barking at the intruder, but ignoring the intruder. Dog's quiet – problem solved!

Many other issues besides immediate pain are also properly dealt with in Chiropractic. Many of the best and most rapid positive outcomes come from Chiropractic care. In the case of injuries: workplace, automobile, or otherwise, it is often wise to see a Chiropractor. I don't recommend skipping emergency care. Serious life or limb threatening injuries naturally require immediate medical attention, but other issues like car accidents without serious bodily damage should make one consider getting an evaluation and probably treatment from a Chiropractor. Whiplash is a very common injury today. Humans aren't built to withstand sudden stops from the unnatural speeds at which we travel in cars.

"He who takes medicine and neglects to diet wastes the skill of his doctors."

Chinese Proverb

Our necks cannot withstand the forces encountered in car accidents where the inertia of your head suddenly meets the resistance of the seat belt. The typical medical regimen her involves pain killers (cover up the warning light) and a neck brace, both of which are not good ideas in the long run, unless you are very severely injured. I've had specialized whiplash training and I know that when you wear a neck brace for extended periods, your neck muscles atrophy at a rate of about 1% per day. That adds up pretty fast in a month or two you could lose half of the strength in your neck. Couple that with painkillers so that you can't tell when you exacerbate your injuries and you're asking for permanent damage. Chiropractic manipulation with other appropriate treatments is a very conservative approach to such injuries that will usually yield excellent results, and it doesn't contraindicate any medical treatment you may need as well.

Worker's Compensation boards are more and more often referring people to Chiropractors for on the job injuries because cost wise and results wise they get more bang for their buck. Employees return to work faster with a lower rate of relapse and better long term results. Another consideration is the fact that Chiropractic care doesn't involve the use of addictive painkillers such as opioids for pain relief, which many states Worker's Compensation programs are trying to minimize. Studies have shown that long term results from Chiropractic care minimize the chances of eventual surgery or permanent disability for workers. A study by BJ Keeney reported by Washington State for those filing Worker's Compensation for low back injuries reported that 42.7% of those who had initial medical intervention eventually had back surgery as opposed to 1.5% for those whose initial treatment was Chiropractic.

> "Sickness comes on horseback but departs on foot."
>
> **Dutch Proverb**

CHAPTER 7

THE FOOD GROUP ILLUSION

For decades, the US government had a simple message on nutrition: "To avoid chronic diseases like diabetes, obesity and heart disease Americans should reduce saturated fat, cholesterol, sugar and sodium."

But today we are sicker than ever. More than 29 million adults in the United States, nearly 9% of the population, are currently suffering from diabetes, according to the Center for Disease Control and Prevention. Obesity has more than doubled since 1980 and fluctuates between 31% and 35%. About half a million Americans die every year from heart disease, which is one in four deaths.

Obviously, we have to change the way we think about food. In 2010, the US Department of Agriculture and the Ministry of Health and Social Services took an important step to resolve the public health crisis by radically changing their dietary habits. They replaced the well-known food pyramid, which has shaped Americans' eating habits for almost two decades, with a new "food plate" that encouraged half of the diet be fruits and vegetables for the first time, while focusing on small portions.

"It's a quick and easy reminder for all of us to know more about the food we eat," First Lady Michelle Obama said when she officially unveiled "the plate" in 2011.

But many experts say these recommendations were not enough to address America's major health problems. Now, as part of a review that takes place every five years, the Government of the United States dietary guidelines are re-examined.

"Diseases of the soul are more dangerous and more numerous than those of the body."

Cicero

For the 2015 Guidelines, scientists and nutritionists urge the USDA and HHS to go further to eat less or avoid completely clearly processed foods.

"I would like the guidelines to move away from nutritional goals and towards real nutrition-based evidence," Dr. Dariush Mozaffarian, Dean of the School of Nutrition and Nutrition Policy at Tufts University.

The first dietary guidelines from 1980 were developed specifically to combat heart disease, which was the biggest recognized enemy of public health at the time. Epidemiological studies dating back to the 1940s and 1950s have linked heart disease to sodium, cholesterol, saturated fat and trans fat. The solution seemed clear: reduce the amount of butter, whole milk, and red meat.

However, as consumers focused on low-fat foods, they generally did not necessarily eat well. "It's not like we're suddenly eating lots of lentils and kale," Dr. David Katz, clinical instructor at the Yale School of Medicine and founding director of the Yale Prevention Research Center. "We replace fats with low-fat junk foods."

The government tacitly approved such products when in 1992 the food pyramid was uncovered. Foods such as bread, cereals, rice, and pasta formed the basis of the pyramid, suggesting that carbohydrates should be the bulk of the diet.

Companies have set themselves to the task of developing low-fat products rich in sugar, starch, and carbohydrates. In the year the food pyramid was introduced, Nabisco introduced its non-fat SnackWell biscuits, which were so popular that grocery stores barely kept them. Similar products followed quickly.

"We get sick because of something inside going wrong!

We get well because of something inside going right!"

B. J. Palmer

"It's true that the focus on fat reduction in the dietary guidelines implicitly leads to higher carbohydrates," said Dr. Walter Willett, chairman of the Department of Nutrition at the Harvard School of Public Health. "And that has become problematic because the vast majority of carbohydrates in the United States are refined and bad for you."

Studies have linked refined carbohydrates to obesity and diabetes, and since the first dietary guidelines were introduced, the rates of these diseases have skyrocketed. Meanwhile, heart disease, the first impetus for the guidelines, remained the number one killer in the United States.

Of course, the guidelines are not responsible for the current health problems of the United States. The unabated promotion of the food industry for unhealthy ready meals and sugary soft drinks also plays an important role. Socio-economic factors make it difficult for many people to access healthy food. And people often ignore healthy diet advice. Still, scientists say it's no coincidence that diabetes and obesity exploded at a time when we focused heavily on eliminating fats from our diet.

The 2010 Dietary Guidelines were the government's first major attempt to address these issues. More importantly, the USDA and HHS have tried to correct Americans' excessive carbohydrate supply by highlighting the importance of fruits and vegetables. While the food pyramid has asked Americans to consume 6 to 11 servings of carbs per day, the new food plate offers a simpler measure: when you fill your plate, you should only consume one-fourth grains and starch. Fruits and vegetables should be half of the plate, and proteins make up the rest.

"People ate a lot more than recommended because we tend to underestimate portions," said Stephanie Dunbar, director of clinical affairs at the American Diabetes Association, about the old guidelines.

"A good laugh and a long sleep are the best cures in the doctor's book."

Irish Proverb

"We underestimated the size of our portions and really did not understand what the 6:00 -11:00 meant." The dish, he said, makes it a lot easier to eat reasonably.

"They've made great progress since 2005," said Dr. Susan Levin, Nutritionist and Director of Nutrition Education at the Medical Responsible Medical Committee, which campaigns for a vegan diet. "They recognize [in the guidelines] that plant-based diets are the healthiest way to eat, and if we could get people to eat that more, we could have a lower prevalence of these chronic diseases."

The new message can do some good. A recent Gallup survey found that a growing number of Americans said they had eaten more fruits and vegetables than in previous years, and many others said they avoided soft drinks and added sugar. Of course, it's not clear if Americans really did change their diets for the better. At least they seem to be more aware of healthy eating habits.

Experts warn however, that the government still has room for significant progress.

For example, the 2010 guidelines suggest that 45% to 65% of calories should come from carbohydrates, a recommendation that some scientists find too vague and confusing. As if the portion sizes were not confusing enough, Americans now have to try to calculate how many calories are in a cereal bowl or on a slice of toast.

New research also suggests that it may be necessary to reconsider our fat mitigation. The 2010 Diets Guidelines found convincing evidence linking saturated fats to high cholesterol and the increased risk of heart disease and type 2 diabetes, the form of the disease associated with obesity and inactivity. However, recent studies suggest that we may lose health benefits in our efforts to avoid the negative effects of fat.

"Water, air and cleanliness are the chief articles in my pharmacopoeia."

Napoleon I

For example, dietary guidelines recommend skimming milk to meet calcium needs while staying below the limits of saturated fat. But some studies show that whole milk can play a role in reducing diabetes risk.

One of the subcommittees working on the guidelines for 2015 plans to discuss saturated fats before September when the group will present its findings.

"We intend to see the latest evidence," said Trish Britten, a nutritionist at the USDA Food Policy and Development Center, who helped manage the 2010 Guidelines and the 2015 process.

Other researchers argue that concentrating on certain nutrients does not address the larger problem of food processing. "It's more important that the meat you eat is not processed in terms of your fat content," said Mozaffarian. "What's more important is what's so much more important, it's sodium and it's cooking, I really want the guidelines to go away from their focus on individual nutrients and fats."

Britten said the 2010 rules have started a new diet-based approach that will continue in the future.

First Lady Michelle Obama, Agriculture Minister Tom Vilsack and then Chief Physician Regina Benjamin reveal the plate of food at the Department of Agriculture in Washington on June 2, 2011.

Obviously, the recommendation that Americans consume healthy, organic and balanced meals is challenging to people at the bottom of socioeconomic leaders who have no Whole Foods in their neighborhood, or who lack the time or money to prepare meals. But nutritional guidelines that promote healthier foods will also improve the diet of the poor.

"The 'i' in illness is isolation, and the crucial letters in wellness is 'we'."

Author Unknown

"Dietary Guidelines are important because they provide information on a range of institutional and government nutrition programs, including school lunches, SNAP policies, and military meals," Willett said, yet, it is a challenge to develop national recommendations for something as individual as health. Researching the latest nutrition and health research and finding studies and interventions for each ethnic, age group and medical need is taxing. Apart from the recommendations on sodium intake, which are broken down by age, race and medical history, government dietary guidelines provide only standardized suggestions.

Specific recommendations on healthy and unhealthy foods can also pit the government against the strong food industry and it's lobbyists.

Food-based policies are "too politically charged," Dr. Marion Nestle, professor of nutrition, food studies and public health at New York University and author of several books on politics in the food industry.

"No industry wants the government to tell people to eat less of their products," Nestle told the Huffington Post. "That's why the" eat more "recommendations refer to food, but" eat less "refers to nutrients."

"While the new guidelines speak freely about foods that are encouraged, the foods they don't recommend are deeply buried in the 95-page report," wrote Caroline Scott-Thomas, a food industry journalist gave them the 2010 guidelines. "Instead, they focus on SoFAS - solid fats and added sugars - a euphemism for many unhealthy foods in our diet."

The USDA has denied that its policies are subject to external pressure.

"There was no impact on the time we were involved in 20 months," Dr. Linda Van Horn, a professor of preventive medicine at the Feinberg School of Medicine at Northwestern University, who was a member of the committee for the Dietary Guidelines 2010.

"How do you make a dimmed light bright again? Remove the interference. How do you increase health in a diseased person? The same way!"

B. J. Palmer

"All industry interests have been completely reoriented, and none of the committee members has anything to do with the food industry.

The food industry, however, has shown that it is more than willing to fight these threatening regulations. In 2011, they launched an intense campaign to defeat the voluntary dietary guidelines for children's food, an effort that has not been completed. And in 2009, the American Beverage Association, Coca-Cola Co., and PepsiCo spent a combined $ 37 million lobbying to help eliminate the federal tax on sugary drinks.

Some health advocates voiced concern that the government's new dietary guidelines, although better, contributed little to the overall health of Americans, given the disproportionate influence of the food industry.

"I've never heard a government telling people to eat more processed foods, dietary guidelines have not told people to drink more soda and eat more cookies," Dunbar said. "There are many determinants of obesity, and it's not just about carbohydrates and fats, there are sociological issues, the food available in the communities and the billions of dollars that promote sweet drinks. "It is very difficult for public health advocates to counter the information generated by this industry," she said. However, experts said they expected the 2015 guidelines to help spread the message about healthy eating habits.

"If they change anything, I hope there is an explicit focus on "Here are the nutritional patterns that make people healthy", "here are the foods that populate those diets," Katz said. really the answer, because if you eat healthy foods in reasonable combinations, you will win. "

"Health of body and mind is a great blessing, if we can

bear it."

John Henry Cardinal Newman

CHAPTER 8

THE INFLAMMATORY SYNDROME - HOW TO COUNTERACT THE EFFECTS OF THIS SILENT KILLER

BATTLING A NEW EPIDEMIC

Now that you are familiar with some of the common factors that wreak havoc on your system, let's now mention what exactly enters your system when influenced or prone to it.

The term "inflammation", is basically an immune reaction triggered by our systems to prevent any infection by bacteria or damage e.g from injuries. If we examine human history itself, we will find out several bacterial infections and disorders that spread to whole populations but people were able to vanish them. Some of these past disorders include, smallpox, influenza, typhoid fever, and bubonic plague, which are almost extinct today.

While the majority of the above bacterial illnesses have almost vanished, nowadays, we have to face a whole new epidemic. There are multiple health issues today that shave off your quality of lives and well-being like such as, breathing problems, memory issues/alzheimer's, allergies, autoimmune disorders, skin problems, and many more. All these issues that especially affect the Western population aren't caused by bacteria like in the past but from inflammation.

In the past two decades, the frequency of degenerative diseases has been constantly on the rise.

"Today, more than 95% of all chronic disease is caused by food choice, toxic food ingredients, nutritional deficiencies and lack of physical exercise."

Mike Adams

Researchers have found that inflammatory disorders have been affecting Americans at an alarming rate because of poor diet habits and induced levels of stress and anxiety. The level of inflammation is at its peak has almost grown to an epidemic. Without any substantial changes to our diet and lifestyle patterns, the country will keep on suffering from diseases like cancer, heart problems, diabetes, Alzheimer's and the list goes on.

WHAT ARE THE EFFECTS OF INFLAMMATION ON THE SYSTEM

When we use the word "inflammation", we usually think of symptoms like "heat", "high temperature", "Irritation", "swelling" and pain somewhere. When a lesion gets inflamed, we can see with our own eyes the inflammation. However, inflammation is not always externally visible like that. The physical signs of "secret" inflammation do emerge but at a much later stage, sometimes when it's too late.

Chronic (long-term) inflammation leads multiple issues in our systems. All sorts of inflammatory disorders may pop up and become a population in our bodies. A person who goes through chronic inflammation, becomes exposed to further health deterioration from diseases and even aging acceleration.

DISORDERS TRIGGERED BY INFLAMMATION

There are various health issues connected with inflammation. Some of the most commonly emerging ones are numerous kinds of arthritis. Arthritis is a broad term that refers to various kinds inflammations in the joint area. Some of the most frequent/common kinds of inflammation-triggered arthritis are:

"It's bizarre that the produce manager is more important to my children's health than the pediatrician."

Meryl Streep

- Rheumatoid arthritis

- Polymyalgia Rheumatica

- Bursitis

- Shoulder Tendinitis

- Gouty Arthritis

Other stressing body problems targeting the bones and joints of our body, that haven't been yet confirmed to be caused by inflammation but they are still under investigation are:

- Osteoarthritis

- Fibromyalgia

- Neck and back pain (in the muscles)

Shockingly enough, the World Health Organization reveals that over 13 millions of people annually lose their lives from cardiovascular disorders. The cancer rates are also alarmingly big, with 8 millions of people losing their lives from cancer annually. Both of these dangerous disorders are caused by chronic inflammation. So in order to control the likelihood of developing such disorders, we must adopt some healthier diet and lifestyle changes.

Heart disorders separately were to blame for 25% of the deaths in the U.S last year and numbers of people affected are constantly on the rise. Almost 50% of the deaths linked to heart disorders were a result of chronic inflammation. The numbers may seem exorbitant and unbelievable but they are shockingly true. Inflammation is a huge factor contributing to heart problems.

"To take in a new idea you must destroy the old, let go of old opinions, to observe and conceive new thoughts. To learn is but to change your opinion".

B. J. Palmer

Based on *National Institute of Health* findings, inflammation is a very vital factor for the development of heart disease and its aggravation. The same goes for other serious and chronic health disorders like cancer and diabetes.

FOODS THAT LEAD TO INFLAMMATION

For those affected by inflammation, diets rich in carbs and low in protein intake can be destructive. As a matter of fact, we've witnessed multiple times that such high carb and low protein diets lead to inflammation while the opposite diet (low carbs/high protein intake), actually keeps inflammation under control and all the negative side effects connected to it.

Every individual organism differs from the other, and thus it is important to spot all the signs and symptoms we experience when we take certain foods. We will offer you a diet against inflammation with all the proper foods to eat later in this report, but at this point, let's delve in a few details.

Processed sugars and foods with an elevated Glycemic Index (G.I), in reality raise insulin levels and trigger an immune system response. There is a communication between inflammatory mediators (prostaglandins, cytokines), and insulin or blood sugar amounts. Studies reveal that when specific stressors emerge, insulin triggers an inflammatory reaction within the system.

Some of the worst foods that trigger an inflammatory response in the body are:

No 1: Sugar/Sweets. High amounts of sugar consumption have been associated with overweight issues, inflammation, and chronic inflammatory diseases like Diabetes Melitus.

"Healing in a matter of time, but it is sometimes also a

matter of opportunity."

Hippocrates

No 2: Typical vegetable oils for cooking and baking. Oils with a high omega-6 fatty acid/low omega-3 acid ratio, also lead to inflammation.

No 3: Trans fats. These fats are typically found on junk food/fast food meals. They are also associated with inflammation, resistance to insulin, and other chronic disorders.

No 4: Non-organic milk and dairy products. Non-organic dairy products can also result in inflammation, especially in the female population, due to the hormones and allergen ingredients they contain.

No 5: Red or processed meat. Eating red and processed meat e.g corned beef cans, is also associated with immune reactions that lead to chronic inflammation within our systems. There is also a clean connection between processed meat consumption and cancer risk, backed-up by many scientific trials.

Other types of foods suspect of causing inflammation are grains/flour, alcohol, synthetic food preservatives, and grain-fed meats. All the above foods should be avoided inf nay signs of inflammation emerge.

LINK BETWEEN STRESS AND INFLAMMATION

Going through chronic emotional, mental, and physical stress affects inflammation in the system to a very high degree. In reality, when the system is exposed stress, cortisol levels start to rise within the body.

Cortisol is specifically a steroid hormone that is produced in response to high levels of stress. This may occur from real stressful events or an unhealthy diet or lifestyle. Concerning inflammation, the stress reaction that starts to develop to relieve the body from tolerating such circumstances isn't switched off. Chronic stress is tied to chronic inflammation responses.

> "The part can never be well unless the whole is well."
>
> **Plato**

In fact, chronic stress has a negative impact on various body functions. For example, it raises blood pressure and hypertension eventually. Chronic blood pressure also puts blood vessels under a tremendous amount of stress. Strokes and heart failures are a common phenomenon in people suffering from chronic inflammation because of inflammatory responses triggered non-stop.

Stress can really "eat" you! Thus, it is vital to learn ways to deal with high stress levels so that you avoid chronic inflammation. Some valuable relaxation methods include:

- Mild exercise

- Yoga/Meditation

- Consuming healthy and nutrient-dense foods

- Learning ways to keep emotional tranquility

- Breathing exercises

INFLAMMATION TREATMENT OPTIONS-THE HARSH ADMINISTRATION OF ANTI-INFLAMMATORY PILLS

The protocol of treatment in response to inflammation is the prescription of anti-inflammatory medicine. The most typically administered drugs in this case are those that provide relief from pain (pain-relievers).

Not long ago, the *American Geriatrics Society* has taken off nearly all non-steroidal and anti-inflammatory drugs from their guide of suggested drugs for people 75+ who experience chronic pain.

"Health is merely the slowest way someone can die."

Author Unknown

It was found out that these drugs are overly prescribed, more than necessary and this may lead to negative side effects on the health of older people. Researchers have found that commonly used pain-relievers like ibuprofen, naproxen, and aspirin are not really beneficial for those going through chronic pain. Due to the research conducted on older subjects, researchers are also seeking to examine the excessive administration of NSAIDS in younger subjects as well.

Anti-inflammatory drugs are aimed to lessen pain and discomfort, minimize swelling, and control inflammation symptoms. They are speculated to help with the development of inflammatory disorder, but they don't always function as intended. Anti-inflammatory substances for pain relief feature NSAIDS such as Ibuprofen and Aspirin. Other substances are the ones called corticosteroids (cortisone, prednisone), and numbing pain relievers.

Typically, anti-inflammatory drug substances demonstrate exaggerated side effects. For instance, the consumption of cortisone for extended periods of time can lead to serious problems with bone strength and integrity. Those experiencing asthma symptoms should also seek an alternative treatment option due to negative side effects from anti-inflammatory drugs. Many chronic takers of NSAIDS also develop stomach ulcers and internal bleeding because of the mucus development blocking attributes of these pharmaceuticals. The gastric wall is further exposed to stomach acid in those who consume NSAIDS for longer periods of time to fight inflammation.

Alternative medicine methods approach the matter of inflammation from another perspective. Instead of prescribing synthetic drugs to hinder inflammatory reactions, they suggest the use of vitamins/nutrients and lifestyle changes. While it's true that some vitamins and nutrients have powerful antioxidant and anti-inflammatory properties, they may not completely eradicate the problem.

"The love you give away is the love you keep".

B. J. Palmer

Alternative medicine adopts a more natural way to treatment of the issue as opposed to taking artificial drugs, but doesn't often consider the trigger cause of inflammation.

Further evaluation needs to be performed to find out the exact leading cause of inflammation. It's not holistic or beneficial to only treat the symptoms, but it's just as important to pinpoint the leading culprit of inflammation.

NSAIDS AND THEIR IMPACT ON INFLAMMATION

NSAIDS (Non Steroidal Anti Inflammatory Drugs) are often prescribed against inflammation. These may differ in power and lasting effects on the system. Prostaglandins are a family of chemical substances released by system cells that trigger inflammation in the system when required.

The enzyme responsible for making these Prostaglandins goes by the name "COX" or (Cyclooxygenase). It is also further divided into 2 enzymes: COX-1 and COX-2. Both of these enzymes trigger the release of prostaglandins which lead to inflammation as a result. NSAIDS actually work to block the activity of such enzymes and control the effects of prostaglandins within the system. This eventually leads to long-term inflammation control. However, prostaglandins that guard the stomach lining and enhance blood clotting are also decreased, which results in stomach ulcers and internal bleeding in the region.

NSAIDS when taken excessively, can interfere with physiological COX-1 activity. NSAIDS also hinder the cyclooxygenase pathways. COX-1 is typically produced by normal functioning. The COX-1 stays stabilized under physiological circumstances. In case an NSAID like Aspirin enters the system, COX-1 becomes acetylated and its arachidonic acid pathway is hindered. The process of acetylation is the culprit behind aspirin's anti-clotting and blood-thinning action.

"By cleansing your body on a regular basis and eliminating as many toxins as possible from your environment, your body can begin to heal itself, prevent disease, and become stronger and more resilient than you ever dreamed possible!"

Dr. Edward Group III

One of the most frequently used NSAIDS is aspirin, which also prevents blood clotting and eventually inhibits strokes and heart failures in people with a heightened risk of experiencing these conditions. NSAIDS though interfere with the physiological activity of heart, kidneys, and stomach due to their action.

INFLAMMATION TESTING-BLOOD EXAMINATION

In those who suffer from long-term inflammation, there is an existing protein secreted by the inflammation region that travels through the bloodstream. One of the common blood tests to find out inflammation is CRP (C-reactive protein test). This test can pinpoint any heightened levels of the protein, which is considered a sign of inflammation.

In several situations when an individual suffers from chronic inflammation which leads to a serious disorder like cancer, arthritis, diabetes, heart failure, or connective tissue (muscle, joints, bones, ligaments) disease, the CRP levels are elevated. These levels are precisely detected through blood testing.

Homocysteine amounts in the blood can also be determined from blood testing. Homocysteine is an acid that is produced by the system physiologically when we consume excessive amounts of red meat. When homocysteine levels are abnormally elevated, the person is a high risk of developing heart problems, atherosclerosis, heart failure, stroke and even Alzheimer's disease.

WHAT'S THE KEY CULPRIT OF INFLAMMATION?

Researchers and medical experts keep on examining the leading cause of inflammation. With so many contributing factors and issues linked to our diets, it's no surprise that gut inflammation has a vital role to play here.

"Early to bed and early to rise, makes a man healthy wealthy and wise"

Benjamin Franklin

We will explain the matter in more details in a later section, but at this point, we should be aware that there is a clear connection between the gut and inflammation. We will examine beyond the natural ways of treating its effects, but study the leading causes behind such symptoms.

Based on scientific evidence, Leaky Gut Syndrome may be the leading cause of many digestive tract diseases like IBS, Crohn's Syndrome, and celiac disease. It can also be the culprit behind the onset of various inflammatory disorders like asthma, allergies, arthritis, and chronic heart problems and disorders.

Practical/holistic medicine takes into consideration the triggering causes of a disorder and doesn't just provide a remedy for the treatment of the symptoms. It is vital to examine all these triggering causes that result in gut and digestive diseases. Gut diseases and syndromes may originate from food sensitivities, leaky gut, and other immunity factors, as stated formerly. We will examine the leading causes in more detail, in a later section.

By addressing inflammation, from a more practical perspective, unlike allopathic or alternative treatment options, we can determine the triggering cause of this modern epidemic. We better know the truth before it's too late!

"Physical fitness is not only one of the most important keys to a healthy body, it is the basis of dynamic and creative intellectual activity."

John F. Kennedy

CHAPTER 9

Eat Your Way Out Of Pain

The anti-inflammation diet

Much of the pain and inflammation an individual suffers is biochemically conditioned.

It makes sense. The pain medication provides relief by affecting biochemistry. Is there a way to naturally influence the chemistry of the body to reduce pain and inflammation? The answer is yes! There are foods that increase inflammation and there are foods that can reduce inflammation. Understanding this will allow you to make lifestyle changes that reduce or even eliminate the number of painkillers you should take.

What is inflammation?

Inflammation is the body's response to an injury. When the tissue is injured, there are a number of chemical changes that occur; we call these changes inflammation. An injured and inflamed body area undergoes a continuous change as the body heals and repairs itself.

When an injury occurs, the body responds with the four features of inflammation: pain, heat, redness, and swelling. Think of a bee sting. First, there is the bite, the initial wound. The body's response to the injury causes redness, heat, and swelling, as well as mild additional pain. The blood vessels in the area of the lesion expand and the white blood cells produce chemicals such as prostaglandins, cytokines, interleukins, and leukotrienes, which cause these inflammatory changes; This happens within 30 minutes of the injury.

"Innate must flow fully, freely, naturally; to, through, and into the educated brain to produce what education calls greatness".

B. J. Palmer

The white blood cells then migrate to the area. If the injury is not too severe, the blood vessels will return to normal within six to eight hours and repair can begin.

What causes inflammation?

Inflammation occurs due to certain chemicals produced by white blood cells in response to an injury. Sometimes there is an exaggerated response to the injury and the inflammation can produce pain that is not proportional to the injury. Medications can inhibit inflammation by disrupting the production of inflammatory chemicals, but they also slow down the healing process. However, they can naturally reduce the inflammation without slowing the healing process.

You may have heard the names of some chemicals involved in inflammation drug advertising. Three examples of these pro-inflammatory chemicals are prostaglandins, cytokines, interleukins, and leukotrienes. Medications that treat allergies and relieve pain and inflammation affect these chemicals. Similarly, diet and supplements can also affect the amount of these chemicals and the inflammation that they produce.

Chemistry of inflammation

The chemistry of pain has been extensively studied. Much of the research involves measuring the number of chemicals involved in the inflammation. Scientists can determine if food can cause inflammation or reduce inflammation by measuring the chemicals produced by inflammation. For example, mice were examined at the University of Buffalo. Mice have been genetically bred to age quickly, have immune system abnormalities, and are prone to developing autoimmune diseases.

"Let food be thy medicine and medicine be thy food"

Hippocrates

In a diet containing omega-3 fatty acids and vitamin E, the mice produced lower levels of vitamin C inflammatory cytokines compared to mice that did not receive omega-3 and omega-3 fatty acids.

Other research has shown that sugar, refined foods, and processed foods can increase the chemicals that cause inflammation. Insensitivity to insulin can lead to inflammation. Insulin insensitivity is the result of too many refined carbohydrates (refined sugars and starch products like sweets, pasta, and white bread). Insulin-insensitive people tend to be overweight and usually carry excess weight in the abdomen, thighs, and buttocks. Studies have shown that overweight people tend to produce more inflammatory chemicals than people who are not overweight.

The fact is the lifestyle you live and the food you eat can affect how much pain you feel. The research appears in the Journal of the American Medical Association

(2004; 292: 1440-1446) shows that the Mediterranean diet can protect the lining of blood vessels and reduce inflammation. In the study, the chemicals that produce inflammation were actually reduced with the diet.

Most diseases are the result of inflammation. Heart disease, Crohn's disease, allergies and even cancer are inflammatory diseases. Controlling the inflammation not only reduces pain but also improves overall health.

A physiotherapist from the Danish Olympic Committee recently conducted a study to document the anti-inflammatory properties of diet and supplementation. This was tested in 1996 for the first time in a group of rowers of the Danish Rowing Association. The study found that a combination of antioxidants and essential fatty acids can be an effective treatment for inflammation in wounds commonly known as "tennis elbow" and "Gulf elbow".

"Just because you're not sick doesn't mean you're

healthy"

Author Unknown

Antioxidants neutralize free radicals. This limits their destructive effects, so athletes should ensure that they receive sufficient levels of antioxidants to protect themselves from stress injuries. Essential fatty acids are important because they promote the production of Type 1 and Type 3 prostaglandins in the body (chemicals that neutralize pain and inflammation)

The amount of antioxidants in your diet is especially important if you want to reduce pain and inflammation. Another aspect of your diet that can reduce pain and inflammation is the type of fats and oils that you consume.

According to a study by Dr. Med. Richard Sperling of Brigham and Women's Hospital can reduce fish oil's inflammatory substances produced by white blood cells. If you have an inflammatory condition such as rheumatoid arthritis (RA), the type of fat in your diet can alter the immune system's inflammatory response.

The intake of polyunsaturated omega-3 fatty acids (PUFA type fish oil) in many industrialized countries is relatively low. Research has shown that increasing the amount of omega-3 fatty acids in the diet different health problems, including atherosclerosis, cardiac arrhythmias, multiple sclerosis, major depression, autoimmune diseases and inflammatory diseases In general, it has been shown that omega-3 PUFAs cause pain in patients with rheumatoid arthritis, inflammatory bowel disease, and other painful conditions.

Anti-inflammatory diet

Much of the pain and inflammation an individual suffers is biochemically conditioned. It makes sense. The pain medication provides relief by affecting biochemistry.

"Those who think they have no time for exercise will sooner or later have to find time for illness."

Edward Stanley

It is logical to think that other ways of influencing the body's biochemistry (such as diet and nutritional supplements) can also affect pain and inflammation. There are foods that increase inflammation and there are foods that can reduce inflammation. Understanding this will allow you to make lifestyle changes that reduce or even eliminate the number of painkillers you should take.

We can use our knowledge about the chemistry of inflammation and develop a diet that really relieves pain and inflammation.

Drink a lot of water every day:

You need water to keep your cells hydrated and protected, to prevent waste, and to ensure the health of your mucous membranes. The most important thing when drinking water when it comes to pain is the fact that water attracts the cartilage and needs enough water for your joints to function properly. Dehydration causes excessive joint wear and may result in disc injury. Drink more water and less soft drinks, coffee, tea or juice.

Eat a lot of vegetables:

Many mean that at least one percent of the food (volume) you eat. Vegetables are very high in fiber, vitamin C, folic acid, antioxidants, and minerals. Some practitioners believe that we do not live on the food we eat; we live on energy in the food that we eat. They believe that raw food is better than cooked food. We will not tell you to avoid hot food, but it is a good idea to increase the amount of fresh and raw foods in your diet. They offer many health benefits such as:

Vegetables are very rich in antioxidants. You may have heard of bioflavonoids or carotenes; these are pigments that give fruit and vegetable color.

"Youth is curious, and success is a game for curiosity seekers. Stay young!"

B. J. Palmer

They are also antioxidants that protect the cells of the solar plant. When consumed, they also provide their cells with antioxidant protection.

A fiber in vegetables reduces the absorption of fats and toxins. Eating enough fiber can help you lose weight and normalize cholesterol and blood pressure.

Vegetables nourish the normal flora, which in turn nourishes the lining of the gastrointestinal tract, produces vitamins and inhibits yeast and other unwanted organisms.

Vegetables accelerate intestinal transit time, reducing gut toxicity and preventing irritation of the gastrointestinal lining.

Vegetables contain folic acid, which is needed to produce serotonin (to prevent depression and overeating), increase energy and reduce the risk of heart attack.

The minerals in vegetables help to prevent osteoporosis. Minerals are also important enzymatic cofactors, so most of the important functions of the body depend on minerals.

Eating vegetables can reduce the incidence of cancer and heart disease, increase energy and mental clarity, reduce the problems caused by intestinal and liver toxicity, and reduce the symptoms of allergies, asthma, arthritis, skin problems, digestive problems, chronic sinusitis pain, and many other health problems,

Ideally, 80% of the volume of food you eat should be vegetables. Corn and potatoes are not considered vegetables. The fruit is good for you as well; it is a good source of vitamin C and fiber. Eating vegetables is striking here because when people are supposed to eat more fruits and vegetables, they tend to increase their consumption of fruits, not the consumption of vegetables.

"If you don't take care of your body, where are you going

to live?"

Unknown

To get well, it is recommended to eat 80% of fresh products (and nuts and raw seeds) and 20% of other foods. Eating four vegetables and two fruits in a food rich in starch and protein meal (proportional to volume) approaches this number. Yes, the instance has 3 ounces of protein per day; you need 12 ounces of vegetables and 8 ounces of fruit per day. You can also get 3 ounces of cereal, but you should not eat it with meat.

The reason why this report works well here is that most Americans tend to eat a lot of grain and protein and not many vegetables. We also tend to combine starch and proteins. Changing these eating habits often has dramatic health effects.

Maintaining health is easier. If you do not have major health problems, you should eat 60% fresh fruits and vegetables, nuts and seeds to maintain your health. This results in one protein, one starch, two vegetables and one fruit. If you have 6 ounces of protein then you need 12 ounces of vegetables and 6 ounces of fruit per day. You may also eat 6 ounces of grain, but you should not eat it with meat. When you eat like this, fruits and vegetables dominate your diet; if they are fresh and raw, much better. If you can get organic products, it will eliminate the stress that pesticides have on your body.

Avoid fried foods, Trans fats, partially hydrogenated oil and hydrogenated oil.

Over time, we find more and worse things about hydrogenated oil and fried foods. Hydrogenation is the way the food industry transforms liquid oils into solid fats. (Trans fat). Although hydrogenated oils are responsible for a variety of health issues, the food industry uses them because they give packaged foods a longer shelf life than if they were made with natural oils. Hydrogenation produces Trans fats that have been linked to a range of health issues, including:

"Healthy is merely the slowest rate at which one can die".

Unknown

The pain and inflammation worsen in patients who consume hydrogenated oils. They chemically prevent the formation of natural anti-inflammatory substances that the body normally produces. If you have chronic pain or recent injury, be sure to avoid hardened oils. In addition, muscle fatigue and skin problems are also associated with hydrogenated oils.

Most chronic diseases are due to inflammation. Because Trans fats increase inflammation, they are also associated with a variety of health problems. Women with a higher Trans fatty acid content in their cells develop breast cancer much more often than women with a low Trans fatty acid content. High Trans fats are associated with coronary heart disease. Lately, much has been written that links inflammation to heart disease. Trans fats are incorporated into cells and make them less resistant to chemicals, bacteria, and viruses. This could be a source of immune system problems. There may be a link between Trans fatty acids and ADD, depression and fatigue. The brain and nerve tissue are fatty. Some researchers believe that trans fatty acids when incorporated into nerve cells affect function and cause problems such as ADD and depression.

Most chips and fried snacks contain hydrogenated oils. Hydrogenated oils are contained in a large amount of packaged foods such as biscuits, cereals, and even bread. They are often found in margarine (margarine is far worse for you than butter); Mayonnaise; and many bottles of salad dressings. Read the labels

All fats are not bad for you.

Permissible fats are raw (not roasted) nuts, extra virgin or extra virgin olive oil and avocados.

"Garbage in garbage out"

George Fuechsel

Avoid refined sugar:

The average American eats 150 pounds of refined sugar a year. Compare that to 17 pounds a year consumed in England in 1750. Refined sugar increases the production of insulin and adrenal hormones and can cause the following health problems. First, sugar increases inflammation. Sugar increases insulin production and insulin can also increase the presence of inflammatory chemicals.

The increased production of adrenal hormones causes the excretion of essential minerals.

Sugar consumption consumes vitamins B and C.

Eating too much sugar aggravates many of the problems associated with emotional stress.

Sugar nourishes the yeast and other single-celled organisms in the intestine that multiply. These organisms produce toxins, irritate the lining of the gastrointestinal tract and replace the normal and beneficial flora, thereby eliminating the benefits of beneficial bacteria.

Eating sugar causes changes in blood sugar levels. The glucose level rises immediately after the consumption of sugar, resulting in insulin production by the body. Excess insulin generates more sugar cravings.

Eating sugar causes insensitivity to insulin. More sugar is consumed; more insulin is produced, etc. This emphasizes the pancreas and sets the stage for adult diabetes.

There is a connection between sugar intake and hypercholesterolemia. Patients with Syndrome X (high cholesterol, high LDL, low HDL and high triglycerides) often have the problem of consuming sugar and refined carbohydrates.

"Throw away your wishbone, straighten up your backbone, stick out your jawbone and go to it".

B. J. Palmer

Sugar can cause or worsen allergies, sinusitis, asthma, irritable bowel, candidates, migraines, fatigue, depression and even heart disease.

Avoid refined carbohydrates:

The average American gets 50% of its refined carbohydrate calories. Refined carbohydrates are grains that have eliminated fiber, vitamin E, B vitamins, bran, and germs. In other words, the nutrients have been eliminated and the strength is retained. They all create the same health problems caused by refined sugar. Go back and read the problems caused by refined sugar and discover that the list of refined starches is exactly the same.

Refined carbohydrates fill up, but not with vitamins and minerals. This highlights your digestive system and your endocrine system. Eating refined carbohydrates consumes valuable vitamins and minerals.

People often eat refined carbohydrates because they are low in fat and falsely think that because they are "complex carbohydrates", they are really good for you. Refined carbohydrates are white bread, white rice, and noodles that are not labeled with whole grains. Read the labels on the bread. Wheat bread with a black bread label is usually not a whole grain. If the label says fortified white flour, you will not get wholegrain. Use brown rice instead of white rice.

Avoid chemical additives:

Avoid processed foods and chemicals. The average American consumes 10 pounds of chemical supplements per year. It had devastating effects on our health. The FDA is testing individual additives, but no one has any idea what additive combinations will do for us. Stay away from foods that are packed with chemical additives and you will be much healthier.

"Life expectancy would grow by leaps and bounds if green vegetables smelled as good as bacon."

Doug Larson

Eat slowly, chew your food thoroughly:

Ideally, chew your food until it is liquid. You will be satisfied with less food and you will have better digestion. Their saliva has enzymes that facilitate digestion. It is also easier to digest small particles than large ones. Do not chew your stress on your digestive system and can lead to poor absorption of nutrients, digestive problems such as flatulence and flatulence, and promote the growth of harmful bacteria in the digestive tract.

Never skip meals:

The omission of meals examines your adrenal glands and therefore can aggravate any inflammatory disease. It can also make you feel tired and eventually gain weight.

If you need more energy or if you have a chronic health problem, you should follow this diet. Although there is a lot of controversy about the alkaline ash content (even for advocates who disagree with the details), patients do well if they follow it. There are some controversial concepts that are added to the basic diet, such as the combination of food and alkaline ashes, but try it. This diet seems to help many health problems.

Summary of anti-inflammatory diet:

Drink a lot of water every day.

Fresh vegetables should dominate your diet.

Avoid fried foods, partially hydrogenated oil and hydrogenated oil.

Avoid refined sugar.

Avoid refined carbohydrates.

Avoid chemical additives.

"Health is a state of complete harmony of the body, mind and spirit. When one is free from physical disabilities and mental distractions, the gates of the soul open."

B.K.S. Iyengar

Eat slowly and chew the food well.

Never skip meals.

If you have a chronic health problem or pain, 80% of your diet should be fresh (fruits, vegetables, nuts, and seeds) and 20% may be other foods (animal products, protein, whole grains). In practical terms, eat four vegetables and two fruits of a starchy food and protein (proportional, by volume).

If you are in good health, save it by consuming 60% fresh produce and 40% other foods (protein, animal products, whole grains, etc.). Specifically, this means one protein, one starch, two vegetables and one fruit (proportional to volume).

If you can, follow some additional rules. Eat mainly raw products. It's good to eat cooked food, but we follow Dr. Reams that we do not live on the food we eat, we live on energy in the food we eat. It is better to eat raw foods than to eat cooked foods. Alcohol and caffeine should be limited.

Do not eat proteins and carbohydrates together. Do not eat fruit with cereals or other foods. It's an old concept called "alkaline ash diet," which is controversial and has written many strange things about it. It turns out that adhering to these two simple rules, along with the rest of nutritional advice, is especially helpful for people with digestive problems.

If you follow the basic diet, you can always follow the eating habits. You can eat meat and potatoes, a sandwich with egg whites and whole grains. The extra discipline of "combining food" is often very helpful for people who are trying to lose weight and have many digestive problems or other health problems. You do not have to limit the amount of food you eat, you just have to change the way you think about food. You really need to think about food by fueling your body and not with likes and dislikes.

218

"In order to change we must be sick and tired of being sick and tired."

Author Unknown

You probably need to plan your meals in advance and not just take food in the race. Try it very strictly for 30 days. Most people can do everything for 30 days. It improves your health and energy and helps you to understand the connection between what you eat and how you feel.

On the next page, we have given you an example of a five-day diet. They are just a few suggestions to help you choose what to eat and not a strict diet. Use it as a guide.

Why not take supplements?

You may have noticed that supplements such as antioxidants and omega-3s have been mentioned in this report. There are even herbs like willow bark, curcumin and others that can naturally reduce inflammation. It is a good idea to seek professional advice before taking supplements. If you take a substance that you do not need, it will not help. The need for supplementation varies from person to person. You can call our office and we can help you with an individual program.

Day 1	BREAKFAST	Apple with almond butter
	LUNCH	Tuna (mix it with olive oil, chopped onion, and celery). Serve it on celery stalks, carrot sticks and/or cucumber slices. You can also include tomato and onion slices
	DINNER	Sweet potato (you can use a small amount of clarified butter--or slice it and cook it in a casserole with sliced apples in pineapple juice), large green salad (oil and vinegar dressing), mixed cooked
	SNACKS	Any fruit, nuts or any vegetable

"Man is a reasoning, very unreasonable manifestation of divine intelligence".

B. J. Palmer

Day 2	BREAKFAST	Oatmeal
	LUNCH	Turkey, large green salad
	DINNER	Brown rice, cooked vegetables, large green salad
	SNACK	Any fruit, nuts or any vegetable
Day 3	BREAKFAST	Quinoa
	LUNCH	Chicken vegetable soup, large green salad
	DINNER	Chicken, large green salad, cooked vegetables
	SNACK	Any fruit, nuts or any vegetable
Day 4	BREAKFAST	Melon
	LUNCH	Hummus, tabouli, goat feta cheese, and cucumber slices
	DINNER	Beef vegetable soup, large green salad
	SNACK	Any fruit, nuts or any vegetable.
Day 5	BREAKFAST	Vegetable omelet (chopped onion, spinach, tomatoes and bell peppers [if nightshades able for you])
	LUNCH	Stir-fried vegetables and brown rice
	DINNER	Broiled salmon, avocado, and a green salad
	SNACK	Any fruit, nuts or any vegetable.

"Health is like money, we never have a true idea of its

value until we lose it."

Josh Billings

CHAPTER 10

THE TRUTH ABOUT STATIN DRUGS

Before we get into more details regarding cholesterol-lowering drugs and the damage they do to our systems, we should first state the status of the big Pharma industry and its connection to your health and cash. There was an extensive study comparing the big Pharma to leading Tobacco industries and the similarities were shocking.

According to various statistics, drugs are the leading cause of death for Americans every year based on *Journal of American Medical Association* findings, along with Tobacco products. The commonalities here are clear in terms of promotion and product placement and both of these industries are literally killing people when their products are used as advertised. Both of these sectors employ underhanded marketing strategies to hide the the truth for the purpose of misleading the audience and authorities appointed to exercise and check compliance with health regulations.

The cover-up or misreporting of scientific studies and evidence has been a common tactic of the big Tobacco industry for many years. We have witnessed the restraint of important studies that expose the damaging or addictive effects of nicotine, for example, or that smoking was directly linked to lung cancer.

A couple of decades ago, in the early 1990s, we were showered with fresh and revolutionary marketing schemes by pharmaceutical companies who showed their ads on TV.

"Time And health are two precious assets that we don't recognize and appreciate until they have been depleted."

Denis Waitley

This was new ground for the industry, and this is where big Pharma and big Tobacco companies are the same. Both industries utilized direct consumer ads to generate demand for their products.

For decades, tobacco companies funded commercial athletics and they still engage in this practice, only in a manner now that doesn't appear as obvious. The big Pharma industry places ads on T.V and radio, and dishes out millions of dollars to influence doctors to use and promote their products on their patients. This is what what we call "lobbying" -- they either pay them cash upfront or fund their holidays, pay their bills, cover their insurance, or provide other indirect benefits. It is common practice to have Pharmaceutical companies sponsor required continuing education, which naturally endorses their own products, at no cost to medical professionals

Many people would be surprised at the level of involvement of big Pharma in the continuing education of Medical Professionals.

Another commonality between Big Pharma and Tobacco is that physicians have a proven history of representing and supporting them. It may be surprising to some, but fifty years ago, doctors were employed as spokespersons of big Tobacco companies and appeared in their ads to promote smoking.

Many doctors are supporters of pharmaceutical drugs and traditional allopathic methods but the new generation of doctors is finally starting to question the adherence to pharmaceuticals as first line treatment of health issues. Some will go beyond the realm of conventional medicine to find effective treatments for their patients. These doctors actually witness their patients improve when not taking any prescription drugs and following other protocols of treatment.

"From the bitterness of disease man learns the sweetness of health."

Catalan Proverb

They do prescribe drugs on occasion, but more commonly as a short-term measure to allow the patient enough time to incorporate lifestyle adjustments and eventually diminish the need for medications.

This, of course, works against the interests of big Pharma as they attempt to make people rely on their drugs as primary healthcare and believe that they need them to stay healthy and ease their symptoms. They go as far to state that drugs are beneficial for you whenin reality, their primary conern is their profits and shareholders. This is why some doctors with a conscience are beginning to separate themselves from the Big Pharma's commercial interests.

Good doctors acknowledge that statin drugs have a short-term role in treating excess cholesterol levels which theoretically impose a serious health risk to that patient. They may prescribe a statin drug for a short period of time, a couple of weeks or few months. Meanwhile, they assist their patients making lifestyle adjustments such as changes to diet habits, exercise, quitting smoking, sleeping enough, and controlling stress. We are going to elaborate on this in a later section.

One of the big issue today with big Pharma is their misreporting and distortion of scientific data and studies regarding statin drugs. This practice was employed by Tobacco industries and the same marketing model was adopted by drug companies recently.

Today we no longer flip magazine pages to see doctors advertising cigarettes, but we do see doctors promoting drugs on T.V and elsewhere. Recently in the news, there was a big controversy over whether grief was a mental health condition that could be treated with prescription drugs or a natural stage of change following the death or the loss of a loved one, or a traumatic event.

"When you get to the end of your rope, tie a knot in it and hang on".

B. J. Palmer

By re-assigning this as a "condition" rather than a natural human process, the medical community is paving the way for pharmaceutical companies to enter and promote their anti-grief/depression drugs to treat it as a condition.

While the American Medical Association may no longer promote tobacco products, they still advertise and endorse prescription drugs that may be harmful or even fatal, and like cigarettes, it may take several years to realize the damage that they do. Pharmaceutical drugs are an incomplete approach to health care as they only address symptoms and can ultimately can be detrimental to health. No one should believe that pharmaceuticals cure health problems. In fact, more prescription drugs usually means more problems with health in the long run.

The medical community doesn't favor change in the status quo of the industry. It is not in their financial interest. They choose to ignore contradictions to this. Their biggest concern is shareholder interests and profit margins. What was once happening in the Tobacco industry, now happens in the Pharmaceutical industry.

Whether referring to the Tobacco or Pharmaceutical industries, similarities are evident. It's all about money. Internal press releases of Pharmaceutical companies report, for example, hundreds of Alzheimer's patients needing to join a drug trial. This is an example of some of the ways they employ to lure people into participation in drug trials.

There is no evidence of any pharmaceutical curing any disease or condition. The exception is insulin which is used to treat Type I diabetes, which is the failure of the body to produce it's own insulin. It's not a cure though, it's treatment. Just as pills may treat pain though, they don't cure the cause of it.

"Health and cheerfulness naturally beget each other."

Joseph Addison

The United States has one of the highest rates of illness and shortened lifespan of the developed world. This in spite of the fact that we consume 60% of the worlds pharmaceutical products. Not only do we suffer from poor health, but we are the most heavy pharmaceutical drug consumers worldwide. We spend so much money on health care, more than any other nation globally, yet our health overall is terrible.

There are no pharmaceutical cures despite what big Pharma would have you believe. Their drugs are just as beneficial as tobacco products. The best they can do is a short-term relief of your symptoms and nothing more. They don't offer any cure which is misleading and the FDA plays a part as well. Now. let's get into some of the issues of statin use.

One of the most common drugs Doctors prescribe is cholesterol control medications. These drugs often go by the name "statins". Statins are used to regulate high cholesterol levels in the blood and are among the most commonly prescribed drugs. Statins mode of action is blocking the compounds that your system needs to produce cholesterol.

The most common statins approved and prescribed in the U.S are the following:

- Lipitor

- Zocor

- Mevacor/Altocor

- Crestor

- Lescol

- Pravachol

"Take care of your body. It's the only place you have to live."

Jim Rohn

Ever since they were released in the U.S market, they quickly became the most commonly prescribed drugs. In the U.S alone, there are between 17-30 million patients that take these drugs.

Despite the fact that statins act as blockers of the production of a particular enzyme in your liver whose key role is to produce cholesterol, this isn't their only mechanism of action. While the do block the cholesterol production enzyme, they also block beneficial enzymes like for example the co-enzyme Q10 which is needed for mitochondrial function.

Health care providers prescribe statin drugs in an attempt to minimize the risk of developing heart problems in a person who shows elevated cholesterol levels. Still, studies demonstrate that statin drugs can actually raise the odds of developing heart disease because they also block the production of coenzyme Q10, which may ultimately result in heart failure. In many cases, patients are advised to take a coenzyme Q10 supplement to compensate for the damage to mitochondria.

Doctor's don't give any credit to the hundreds of studies and evidence that show a link between statin drugs and heart problems. Not only do people consuming statin drugs raise the chance of inflicting damage to their mitochondria, they also expose themselves to other health concerns like cancer, diabetes, nervous system issues, mood disorders, and of course heart problems. We are going to elaborate on this further in another section.

THE HARSH TRUTH ABOUT STATINS

In the U.S separately, 1 out of 4 people 45+ year old, are users of a cholesterol regulating drug. Physicians are giving statin drugs to people that are obese, follow bad diets, or don't do any form of physical activity and have high cholesterol levels.

"Your body is a temple, but only if you treat it as one."

Astrid Alauda

During the 60s, there were only a handful of nonconformist scientists and researchers in the medical profession and in the emerging natural health food act that believed that Cholesterol was an issue. Most doctors didn't pay much attention unless cholesterol levels exceeded 300. Recently, the anti-cholesterol fuss is virtually impossible to overlook and the medical care industry proceeded to acknowledge the issue of high cholesterol. Today, any levels exceeding 250 are deemed a concern. Today people are advised to stay away from red meat, dairy and eggs due to their cholesterol content and potential link to heart problems.

Now it wasn't initially the medical industry that made cholesterol into an issue, but the food processing industry. The food processing industry dished out billions of dollars to promote their own propaganda to mislead the U.S public, but the Big Pharma industry kept on turning a blind eye to this perceived cholesterol issue.

Until statin drugs were invented. Even though cholesterol has been demonized, the medical industry attempts to exorcise this "demon" that lives within us by telling us to avoid meat and eggs.

This fight against the cholesterol has been going on for 25 years. Over the last few years, there have been many new studies claiming that cholesterol was never the true culprit of heart disease. Still, statins, the drugs used to regulate cholesterol levels do have have a large effect on various body functions. We will study this in more depth as we proceed in this report. Let's examine now all the possible risks of statins.

STATINS AND CANCER CONNECTION

There are series of studies carried out examining the link between statin drug consumption and cancer risk. There was one study conducted during 2005-2008 consisting of 400 men who suffered from Prostate cancer.

"Everything comes to him that waits" — But here is one that's slicker: The man who goes after what he wants, gets it a darn sight quicker.

B. J. Palmer

The study's purpose was to find out whether there was a connection between statin drugs and a risk of developing prostate cancer. Conductors of the study examined 400 male patients who were initially diagnosed with prostate cancer during the 3 years of the study. In short, the study found out that those who took statin drugs (any levels) were linked to an elevated prostate cancer risk. What's more surprising is that the odds rose more as the dosage of statin consumption increased. In other words, the more statins the patient would consume, the greater the odds of developing prostate cancer. Based on this study's findings, they have concluded that statins may possibly elevate risk of developing cancer.

While the findings still appear to be inconclusive--some studies show a higher risk, some lower, and some no clear connection between the two. But what we can tell, is that conventional medicine still fails to acknowledge and study the complications of unnaturally trying to minimize cholesterol levels--they simply have no idea, or ignore whether the consumption of such drugs may raise chances of developing cancer. This is discouraging news.

With so many millions using statin drugs, they are unknowingly part of the large experiment of cholesterol-regulating drugs and have no real clue of what really goes on inside their bodies.

More than a decade ago, studies had shown that besides decreasing cholesterol levels, statins could possibly encourage the development of new blood vessels. This occurrence could help avoid any cardiovascular problems e.g heart failure but at the same time, it could also encourage the formation of cancer tumors. Other researchers have found exact opposite findings.

"Mainstream medicine would be way different if they focused on prevention even half as much as they focused on intervention…"

Anonymous

Alternative and independent studies demonstrate that statins can suppress angiogenesis (blood vessel formation) and therefore, we can't really claim that statin safety and effectiveness is backed-up by solid scientific research. The findings are contradictory. So what or whom we should believe?

The link between statin drug use and cancer goes further back than these previous studies. In 1996, a report published on the *AMA Journal* had found that all kinds of the most commonly used cholesterol lowering drugs (fibrates and statins) triggered cancer in mice. They added that prolonged clinical studies and a thorough marketing monitoring process should be held over the next few decades to find out whether cholesterol drugs trigger cancer in humans. Finally they suggested that until this happens, the findings from any study suggesting that any cholesterol lowering drugs are beneficial, should be avoided excluding patients that possess a high risk of developing coronary heart illness.

More recently in 2008, there were more studies carried out and findings showing a strong connection between statins and extremely elevated risks of developing cancer and cancer-associated deaths in patients who took the cholesterol regulating drug called "Inegy/Vytorin". The drug is a mix of the famous statin called "Simvastatin" and another drug called "ezetimibe". This drug essentially stops the absorption of cholesterol in the gut.

The drug demonstrated its ability to decrease LDL cholesterol levels by a significant 61% , which should bear a positive impact on cardiovascular function, based on the leading theory that elevated levels of LDL are linked to an elevated risk of developing heart disease. Yet there was no evidence that there was any good net effect on the main outcome (e.g cardiovascular problem reduction) while more patients developed cancer while taking the drug (105 users as opposed to 70 placebo) and more cancer-associated deaths.

"Our bodies are our gardens – our wills are our

gardeners."

William Shakespeare

Many months following the study, the outcome of these findings were published by the *American Academy of Cardiology* which stated that this heavy drug combo should only be taken as a last resort and there is no data supporting that Ezetimibe, which decreases cholesterol levels, improves clinical results such as heart failure risk.

A year later and in December 2009, the U.S FDA intervened and announced completion of their study concerning the drug and its outcomes. They announced that in other clinical reviews it was found that it was highly improbable that the drug Vytorin or Zetia could elevate the risk of developing cancer.

Since there are no solid scientific findings, the FDA generated an announcement. It's hard for us to believe FDA statements as they has been proven false many times.

BONE AND MUSCLE ISSUES RELATED TO STATINS

As mentioned earlier, it is an irony that the main purpose of prescribing statins is to minimize the risk of developing cardiovascular problems as there is evidence suggesting that they may actually raise the risk of developing heart problems because they suppress the production of the beneficial Q10 coenzyme. This suppression could eventually lead to heart failure. But the damaging effects of statins do not stop here--they also have a damaging effect to the myoskeletal system as well.

Issues with the muscles and bones, strains, pain/discomfort have been linked with cholesterol-regulating statins. Even though the pain is sometimes extreme, its is often misdiagnosed as something else. A typical side effect of statin drugs is myalgia (pain in the muscles) and most physicians fail to recognize this.

"The best and most efficient pharmacy is within your own

system."

Robert C. Peale

The most common misdiagnoses people are given for this condition are: bursitis, tendinitis, tendinopathy, rotator cuff syndrome and others. There are even known incidents of patients undergoing surgery for suspected rotator cuff syndrome or other myoskeletal problems that didn't actually exist.

Based on *British Medical Journal* statements, muscle deterioration and myopathy have been noticed in 11 out of 100K patients taking statins. The pain is experienced as fatigue, weakness, and muscle strain and can start as a feeling of discomfort that gradually increases. These symptoms can negatively influence a person's mobility and daily schedules.

Statins have been linked with rare occurrences of extreme myopathy and rhabdomyolysis along with inductions of creatine kinase, proteinuria (excess protein in urine) and renal failure. Coordinate usage with gemfibrozil, cyclosporine, niacin and erythromycin or azole antifungal compounds may raise the risk severity of myoskeletal symptoms. Other factors linked with an elevated risk of statin-triggered myopathy feature aging, small body physique, being a female, experiencing liver or renal issues, hypothyroidism and diabetes type I and II.

In rare instances, statins can trigger a life-threatening pathological condition known as *rhabdomyolysis* which may trigger kidney or liver failure and death. This is a very rare occurrence happening to 3.4 patients out of 100K. Rhabdomyolysis has been documented more in those who use statin drugs along with other drug combos like gemfibrozil. This is fact that the medical industry fails to acknowledge.

Another issue for patients who take cholesterol regulating medications like statins suffering from myoskeletal issues is raised serum CPK (Creatine Phosphokinase) which demonstrates muscle tissue breakdown. In extreme circumstances, muscle necrosis (death of muscle tissue) can result which leads to excessive CPK flooding the kidneys.

"An optimist is the one who sees a light where there is none. A pessimist is one who blows it out".

B. J. Palmer

As stated earlier, statin drugs inhibit the release of coenzyme Q10, which poses a very critical health hazard. As the system becomes more and more drained of this vital enzyme, those using statin drugs will often experience tiredness, weakness, muscle strain, and in rare occasions heart failure. Coenzyme Q10 plays a major role in the procedure of neutralizing free radicals and the optimal generation of energy within the cells.

Sadly, most people using statins drugs do not know that they also need Q10 and doctors who should know this, don't commonly advising supplementation of the enzyme. In the U.S. alone, it is very rare for a physician to prescribe both of these to prevent any potential side effects to cell mitochondria. It is beneficial to take Q10 during the beginning of statin use.

It is vital to bear in mind when using a statin drug to use a coenzyme Q10 supplement (even if your doctor doesn't tell you to do so). If you are 40+, it is highly suggested that you take this in ubiquinol form. This is the most efficient and bioavailable form of Q10 with a broad range of health benefits. There are some studies showing its potential to decrease the risk of developing Alzheimer's disease, Parkinson's, and even cancer as well as early aging by slowing down the shrinkage of telomeres which can retard the process of aging.

Unlike prescription pharmaceuticals which are deadly for more than 125K Americans annually, there are no documented side effects of Q10 supplementation and no evidence of anyone dying from taking it. There is also currently no evidence suggesting any potential negative impacts arising from its use.

"Health is not simply the absence of sickness."

Hannah Green

Dr. James W Zielinski DC

PROBLEMS WITH THE NERVOUS SYSTEM

The nervous system is also affected by the use of cholesterol-regulating drugs like statins. There are some documented cases of memory problems linked with Simvastatin. In these occasions, individuals eventually developed memory problems over time while using statin drugs. Once these people stopped using statin drugs, their memories returned within 30 days.

Some folks suffering from memory loss also complain about a failure to keep their focus and fear they are starting to show early symptoms of Alzheimer's disease when using statins.

Earlier studies also link statins with an elevated risk of developing delirium (sudden confusion state) after surgery . University of Toronto researchers examined patient data of 284.000 patients after surgery. Delirium is frequently undiagnosed in these patients, but researchers estimate that in around 10% of all surgeries, patients experience delirium episodes and in 13% of the patients who use statins. Since delirium episodes can slow down recovery, this is big problem. The theory behind this issue is that statins trigger blood flow to the brain, adding strain to the heart, although there is no solid evidence that this is the case. The researchers affirmed that more studies and trials need to be done to address these serious concerns regarding surgery and the use of statins and their effect on nervous system health and function in the long run.

Some of the most frequent negative side effects linked with statin drugs are headaches, dizziness, and cognitive deterioration. Additional nervous system side effects associated with the use of statin drugs feature trembling, vertigo, lightheadedness, memory problems, peripheral nerve damage, cranial nerve impair and delusions. These issues are major and shouldn't be neglected, yet they are often overlooked by medical professionals, pharmacists and big Pharma.

"My own prescription for health is less paperwork and more running barefoot through the grass"

Leslie Grimutter

We have already discussed the effects of statin drugs in myoskeletal system. These two systems are connected to each other and they are both influenced by drugs. Muscle fatigue and neuropathy are linked with each other.

People say that things get on their nerves. Statins are not the first thing that we can think of, but they certainly do get on our nerves. Studies reveal that 1 out 10 patients taking statin drugs suffer from a mild to extreme case of neuropathy. Symptoms include muscle fatigue, struggle when trying to rise up from a bed or chair, breath problems, problems with movement and walking and more.

WHAT BIG PHARMA DOESN'T TELL YOU

While statin drugs do work in decreasing "bad" cholesterol (LDL) in our blood, it is important to assess that they are various sizes of LDL compounds. The LDL compound size does matter as this is often blocked, leading to inflammatory responses. Sadly, this fact is not related and very few people are aware of it. Big Pharma really doesn't tell you the truth that statins can't regulate the size of the cholesterol molecules.

The only way to ensure that your LDL particles are big enough to avoid getting blocked and trigger inflammation is by changing your diet. Ideally the size of LDL particles is regulated by Insulin. If you follow a diet that keeps insulin levels balanced and optimal, then everything will run smoothly. The LDL particles will change and won't trigger inflammation.

Instead of worrying about your cholesterol levels, people should do things that minimize inflammation. Inflammation often has the following culprits:

"The best doctor gives the least medicine."

Benjamin Franklin

- Oxidized cholesterol (cholesterol that become tainted e.g from overcooked eggs)

- Consumption of sweets and grains

- Consumption of trans fats (from processed food)

- Inactive lifestyle

- Smoking

- Stress/anxiety

The biggets factor that contributes to the development of heart disease is following unhealthy lifestyle habits. A diet filled with unhealthy trans fats from junk food, sweets, sodas and lack of physical activity is really what fuels the problem and not cholesterol. A clean and healthy lifestyle keeps the system functioning the way nature intended. Statins are very commonly prescribed drugs as evidenced by the millions of people using them. Last year only, more than $13B was spent on the two most popular statin drugs. This implies that people are buying these drugs at alarminglyhigh rates. Based on the latest research findings, Americans spend 3X more money in drugs than other nations yet suffer from poor health and shorter life spans. But ultimately, we are all accountable for our own well-being. With a little education we can protect ourselves from harm. Don't give in to the commercials telling you that their new cholesterol regulating drug will improve your cardiovascular health and save you from heart failure. It's all lies.

Consider all the risk parameters and find out the truth by yourself. Don't allow Big Pharma to tell you what to take. The truth could save your life!!

A "specialist" is one who knows more and more about less and less".

B. J. Palmer

CHAPTER 11

A Reasonable Approach to Exercise

As we specified earlier, exercise is just as vital as diet. We also specified in an earlier section that proper exercise can do wonders for your posture. In this chapter we will touch briefly on the benefits and performance of exercise in a complete health regemin. There are entire books dedicated to this subject, and it is only a fraction of the scope of this book, so we will not get to far in depth.

We should also discuss the influence of exercise in various functions of the body and specifically the brain and circulation.. We are familiar with the concept that the harder you exercise, the better you'll feel. But do you know why is this the case? Exercise actually makes your brain function better. When you exercise you also release endorphins, "reward hormones", and increase blood circulation.

Motivation is key to successfully implementing an exercise program into your life. There is a great article by Vicky Pierson and Renee Chloe called "The Motivation To Move" that provides some pretty handy tips on motivation. They specifically mention 3 types of factors that affect exercise motivation. These feature individual factors, regime factors, and environmental parameters.

When assessing your individual factors, ask yourself the following questions:

"The doctor of the future will no longer treat the human frame with drugs, but rather will cure and prevent disease with nutrition."

Thomas Edison

- What are your feelings on the exercise's value?

- What previous exercise experience do you have?

- What levels of skills do you possess for the exercises you have picked? Are these too challenging for you based on your skills?

- Where are you when it comes to motivational status?

- Do you find the exercise to be very challenging or painful?

- Are you able to tackle any obstacles that hinder your exercise success for example health, work, traveling time and other time restrictions, so that you are able to follow your exercise regime?

- Does your exercise regime fit your schedule?

- Does your chosen exercise plan need some kind or preparation/set-up to be implemented? Nothing kills motivation more than having to spend energy and time for setting up.

- Is your program varied enough so you are not bored but aren't pushing yourself too hard either?

- Does the regime allow for flexibility and variation to keep your interest intact?

Then we'll look at environmental factors.

- Do you feel comfortable with the location where you exercise? For example, some females may be uncomfortable with the idea of going to exercise in health clubs if they have a reputation of being pick-up spots. Obese folks may also feel embarrassed when comparing themselves to other more fit people in the gym.

"Our health is something we often take for granted. But, there are some things in life that should never be taken for granted. Take care of yourself."

Catherine Pulsifer

- Have you arranged some signals to help remind you to exercise such as hanging your gym back by your door.

- Can you still exercise regardless of environmental conditions? What are your backup options when you exercise outside?

- Do you have a support mechanism? One good way to keep motivated is getting family members or friends to join you.

This article also recommends some additional tips to keep your interest and motivation intact:

- Acumulating your progress. You can start with smaller targets first and then work your way up to bigger ones.

- Seeking a good example/role model who also was in similar position as you when they started.

- Being realistic with yourself. Don't try to run a mile if it beyond your capabilities--start walking around your neighborhood first. Then run a bit farther next time and so on.

Additionally:

- Set short term goals and pat yourself in the back for reaching them

- Allow for diversity in your fitness schedule. You don't want to become bored as progress. Then, incorporate more varied exercises as you go through your regime.

- Concentrate on the benefits of getting fit.

- Manage your time smartly. There is no need in spare a great deal of time to reach your goals.

"The man who earns a million but destroys his health in the process is not really a success"

Zig Ziglar

- Be aware of your restrictions and remain just above your comfort zone. Of course, you will need to acknowledge your limits. The better you know yourself and what you are capable of doing, the better your chances of success.

We have previously mentioned the effects of exercise on your brain. When you start a tense workout, jogging, or even walking, there are some interesting reactions on your brain activity. A 2010 study conducted by the University of Pittsburgh has shown that ongoing exercise enhanced cardiovascular activity and circulation of oxygen to all cells and of course, the brain. The more oxygen gets into the cells, the healthier the cell becomes.

The study showed that people who engage in frequent jogging or walking programs have shown greater grey matter expansion and brain integrity. The people who exercised demonstrated a decrease in overall stress levels, depression, and anxiety because of increased grey matter.

When we talk about the nerve cell connections, we include chemicals secreted in the brain called 'neurotransmitters'. There are billions of brain cells that interact with one another by way of neurotransmitters. It is the neurotransmitter production that allows interaction and signalling between the brain cells. Exercise raises neurotransmitter levels and creates a positive mood and feelings of well-being. Feelings of bad mood or stress can be counteracted by the heightened release of neurotransmitters.

When someone begins to exercise, the brain produces a cocktail of various neurotransmitters like Dopamine, serotonin, and endorphins. Serotonin is made from the amino acid "L-Tryptophan" in brain nerve cells. It is produced in three regions of the body: the intestinal tract, expanded blood cells, and of course the nervous system.

"Keep your head cool — feet warm — mind busy. Plan work ahead and stick to it — rain or shine. If you are a Gem, someone will find you".

B. J. Palmer

When someone begins to exercise, even for a few consecutive days, the levels of serotonin in the system start to rise. Exercise also helps trigger the production of L-tryptophan which in turn raises the levels of dopamine in our system. Dopamine is another kind of brain neurotransmitter which increases during exercise. Dopamine, as is backed-up by numerous scientific studies, is responsible for enhancing motor coordination and function as well as muscle recall. By exercising, we help our system release more serotonin and dopamine.

Just 30 minutes of exercise is enough to trigger the production of dopamine and serotonin. We can also decrease stress and promote a more pleasant and happy mood. The endorphins that are triggered from physical activity by the pituitary gland, can also help control stress and body fatigue. Endorphins attach to receptors in the brain referred to as "opioid receptors". When these are blocked the production of neurotransmitters is paused and this slows brain impulses. Endorphins therefore reduce stress.

While physical activity yields many benefits for our grey matter it is also beneficial to other regions of our brains such as the cerebellum. This is a region in the brain that enables us to coordinate our physical movements such as picking up the spoon or using a keyboards or balance.

The cerebellum plays a role in:

- Balance of movements

- Muscle coordination

- Muscle timing

- Posture balance

"Health is the condition of wisdom, and the sign is cheerfulness, - an open and noble temper."

Ralph Waldo Emerson

The cerebellum gets signals from numerous regions of the spinal cord and brain in order to coordinate the above activities. It is the composition of this little brain region that makes it act the way it does during exercise and physical activity.

Below are some exercises which can help your cerebellum and improve muscle coordination and balance:

1. While standing still, hold up one leg while clapping your hands together over your head. Repeat 20-30X. You can also shut one eye and switch between your eyes while performing this exercise.

2. While standing still, hold up your arm over your head while holding up your opposite e.g left hand, right leg. Repeat 20X.

3. Perform around 10 latches while holding up your arms sideways. Repeat 10 times before switching your legs.

By performing the above exercises for your cerebellum, you can improve your muscle power, coordination, balance and accuracy of movements. As the cerebellum gets certain signals from your sensory functions your muscle coordination will improve.

Exercise enhances the activity of cerebellum. When you do exercises that are specifically targeted to the cerebellum, it improves communication between the motor and sensory systems. The cerebellum isn't just an inactive receiver when it comes to getting sensory signals. The cerebellum's duty is to get signals and then translate what parts of the sensory information are needed for the coordination of movements. Exercise enhances the function of cerebellum.

"Alternative Medicine is now much bigger that what anyone can think, and it plays a role in health and human welfare beyond what anyone could have imagined a decade ago."

Dr. Johnson C. Philip, Alternative Medicine And Arthritis

Apart from influencing the brain and neurotransmitters, exercise also affects hormonal function, mood, and other areas of the body. For enhancing muscle mass, burning fat, and balancing cholesterol levels, one should exercise frequently and follow a healthy diet.

The pituitary gland, located in the frontal lobe of the brain, is responsible for producing testosterone, which in turn triggers the production of muscle protein. The hypothalamus secrets growth hormone, which in turn enhances muscle recovery and immune system function/regeneration. Another noteworthy hormone is cortisol, which is released by the adrenal glands when the body experiences stress. Elevated physical fatigue translates to higher cortisol levels. Cortisol has the opposite function of testosterone as it relaxes and breaks down tissues as opposed to enhancing them.

Cortisol slows down protein production, enhances the conversion of protein to energy, and controls tissue expansion.

While it doesn't help with building muscle, it is important in managing inflammatory reactions and even out blood glucose levels during times of fatigue. Exercise may cause fatigue and this is why cortisol is secreted. However, due to the release of other neurotransmitters, like dopamine and serotonin, production of cortisol is controlled. Additionally, weight and strength training increases the amounts of other hormones and this also halts the production of cortisol.

Other functions that are positively influenced by exercise are the cardiac and thyroid function. Exercise is vital for a strong heart. Doctors have preached this for ages and the *American Heart Association* confirms it. Cholesterol levels are decreased because of raised cardio exercise and the general function of the heart gets better.

"Health is the greatest gift, contentment the greatest wealth, faithfulness the best relationship."

Buddha

Doctors are not able to tell the exact mechanisms and links between exercise and heart health, but studies carried out by the University of Texas medical center, show that there is a definite link between the two. Exercise facilitates the burning of fat in those who are obese may have higher LDL levels in their blood. LDL in particular is the "bad" cholesterol that is often to blamed for heart problems. We will discuss the truth about cholesterol later. Exercise is considered to trigger the production of enzymes in the blood and carry LDL from the blood to the liver. The liver then gets it and expels it out of the system.

The thyroid gland is also positively influenced by frequent and mild exercise. Exercise activates a sluggish metabolism and helps to decrease insulin levels. This is why endocrinologists suggest exercise to boost underactive thyroid function.

Exercise supports metabolic processes and gets your system going. It also helps release hormones in the body which are necessary for the thyroid to function properly. For the purpose of decreasing insulin and enhancing general health, physical exercise is vital.

Mood is also influenced by exercise. As we mentioned earlier, when exercising, dopamine and serotonin are released in the brain. Serotonin boosts mood and raises feelings of satisfaction and fulfillment. Serotonin levels are elevated in the system after a vigorous exercise regime. This of course is very beneficial in combating stress, depression, and fatigue.

Endorphins do wonders in the body by functioning as pain relievers. They also control the physical strain linked with exercise enabling you to work harder. There is a reason why marathon runners state that any chronic pain they have suffered previously, was lessened during running or any other form of physical activity. Endorphins in a few words can help alleviate any pain and ease your comfort during exercise so you can go on. Endorphins are responsible for the "runner's high".

"There is a power within — a fountain head of unlimited resource — and he who controls it controls circumstances instead of it controlling him".

B. J. Palmer

Dopamine also affects mood and is secreted by the brain--when its levels are balanced, it helps regulate good and quality sleep patterns. Dopamine also acts in conjunction with serotonin; when the latter is depleted and dopamine is raised, serotonin raises as well.

Adrenaline is also raised short-term during vigorous exercise. Adrenaline is a neurotransmitter secreted by the adrenal glands. When exercise intensity is high, neural signals get sent to the adrenal glands. This leads to the release of adrenaline. The heart rate and pressure is elevated and the sympathetic nervous system is activated. When exercising, adrenaline levels also offset sensations of stress and fatigue.

Exercise is vital for optimizing the brain and body functions. The whole body requires exercise to work at its peak. Circulation is also exercise dependent. Your heart pumps blood out, but it has no mechanism to pump it back. This is done by physical exercise. Your arteries are the vessels which carry blood away from the heart, but the blood is brought back in veins. The difference is that your veins have uni-directional or one-way valves built into them that only allow blood to flow in one direction. The mechanism that propels it is muscular contraction, which squeezes the veins and moves the blood to the next chamber. This occurs all along the length of the vein and the action of your muscles moves the blood along, chamber by chamber, until it returns to your heart. Vericose veins are the result of these chambers failing, and blood pooling in them, either by means of the valve malfunctioning, or insufficient muscular contraction. Therefore, physical exertion is vital to complete circulation, as it is the mechanism of propelling blood back to the heart.

"If you want to dramatically improve your self-esteem the one sure way to do this is to get very, very fit."

Christopher Quinn